CANCER & COSMETICS

Combinations That Can Hurt You

A Guide to the Safe Use of Salon and
Cosmetic Treatments for the Cancer Patient

RACHEL FURMAN, RPh.

CRF PUBLICATIONS

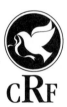

CRF PUBLICATIONS
11684 Ventura Boulevard
Studio City, CA 91604
www. rachelfurman.com

Printed in the United States of America.

ISBN 0-9701114-1-8

Order from CRF Publications or by visiting our website at www.rachelfurman.com

CONTENTS

CHAPTER THREE: SKIN CANCER

To My Friends, the Aestheticians,

As those of you who have read my first book, *Drugs and Cosmetics: Combinations That Can Kill You,* or heard me lecture know, I have been alarmed for some time about the lack of knowledge of basic chemistry, physiology and biology I encounter out in the field.

This is not your fault. Few states require classes in these subjects as part of your training. Unfortunately, you are still ethically, morally, and legally responsible for the results of the treatments you administer.

Did you know that some common salon treatments can actually encourage the spread of certain cancers? Most aestheticians don't. No one wants to be responsible for spreading cancer. No aesthetician wants to do deadly harm to her clients. But it happens. Everyday. Why? Some aestheticians just don't know any better.

That's why I wrote this book. It will not make you an expert in providing salon treatments to cancer patients, but it will make you more aware of what NOT to do. It will give you the one tool you need to make safer decisions. If you don't read another sentence in this book, read the next one. **CALL THE TREATING PHYSICIAN BEFORE YOU ADMINISTER ANY SALON TREATMENT TO A CANCER PATIENT, A RECOVERING CANCER PATIENT, OR A FORMER CANCER PATIENT.**

If you don't think you have clients that fall into these categories, think again. 192,000 new cases of breast cancer are diagnosed every year. A staggering 42,000 women die of this cancer every year! It is the second leading cause of death from cancer after lung cancer and is the leading cause of death in women aged 40 to 55. You have clients that have, have had, or will have cancer. The more you know about how to treat and support them, the better job you will be able to do.

I hope you find the information in this book helpful. At the end of the book is a list of other sources about cancer. The solution is knowledge. You can never have too much of it.

Yours,

Rachel

CHAPTER 1

What is Cancer?

What is cancer?

The medical term for cancer is malignant neoplasm: neo meaning new and plasm meaning growth. Cancer is a common term that describes a large group of diseases. The common thread is an uncontrolled rapid spread of cells that, if untreated, will take over the body and eventually cause death.

There are more than 1.22 million new cases of cancer diagnosed every year. This number is evenly divided between men and women. After heart disease, cancer is the second leading cause of death in the United States. More than a quarter million women.die every year from cancer. Most cases occur in people over the age of 65, making age the largest risk factor for cancer.

Breast cancer is the most prevalent cancer in women, comprising 30% of all cancers. But the biggest killer is lung cancer, claiming 25% of all female deaths.

Although the treatment of cancer has advanced tremendously and survival rates have been increasing constantly, society's perception of cancer is different from that of diseases like diabetes or heart disease. The fear of finding out one has cancer prevents a lot of people from doing the one thing that can save their lives: going to the doctor for a check up.

People experience a wide range of emotions when diagnosed with cancer. The most common one is fear: fear of treatment, fear of the loss of the ability to function, fear of the change in physical appearance and fear of death. People diagnosed with cancer also experience anger, frustration, denial, loss of control, confusion, grief, loneliness, isolation and depression.

Why does a person get cancer? This is a question that has no definite answer. What is known is that it takes a long time for the cancer to evolve and that a multitude of mistakes, or in scientific terms, mutations, need to happen inside a cell to make it abnormal. Cancer can be viewed as a chain of uncorrected mistakes in the information center of the cell. At least 5 to 10 mutations are needed to cause enough damage to the cell for it to become cancerous. These changes occur in the DNA, the cell's information center. The DNA is the blue print of the cell's functions. It defines what type of cell the cell is, how long it will live, what type of substances it needs to produce, and when and how often it should divide. Every cell has built-in controls that regulate and repair cellular "mistakes". The body also has regulators which help with the controls. These regulators are called the immune system.

The DNA is also called the genetic imprint. This is the information that was passed to us from our parents and grand parents. We will pass it on to the next generation and so on and so on. The genetic information in the cell is the part that gets damaged. This is why cancer is considered to be a genetic disease. With that said, it is different than an hereditary disease. Hereditary means that if your parents had it, you will get it. With cancer it's the fact you have inherited the gene that makes you susceptible to the disease, but that susceptibility does not mean that you will get it. It only means that you have the potential. There are many cases of identical twins where one got cancer and the other did not. So what makes the difference? The environment.

The environment is a major risk factor for cancer. In this discussion the term environment represents all the other factors that are present in a person's life, for example, where ones lives. In Los Angeles the air is polluted making it more likely that a person living there will get lung cancer than a person living in Colorado Springs. Another example is a person living in Australia has a higher risk of developing skin cancer than his friend who lives in Sweden. Smoking and alcohol are other negative environmental factors.

Diet is another factor. Although it is hard to research we know that women in Asia have almost no incidences of breast cancer and yet the same women, when adopting a western diet, have the same cancer risk as their western counterparts.

On the other end there is no scientific proof that vitamins, minerals, anti-oxidants, herbal remedies or food supplements in any amounts larger than are present in normal food intake can prevent cancer.

Stress, although not clearly identified in the medical literature, has a major negative influence on the immune system.

Age is another important factor. Statistically, the older the woman, the more likely she is to get cancer. It can be explained in the context of machines. Our body is a very complicated machine. With use, every machine suffers from wear and tear. So does the body. When the body is young and the machine is new, it can absorb the bumps in the road, but there comes a point when the machine gets worn out. The older the machine the more likely it is to break down.

Carcinogens present another environmental threat to the body. These are substances that have the potential to change the cell's DNA and cause it to malfunction, turning it into a cancerous cell.

All cancers start with one cell. In order for the cell to become a cancer cell it needs to be able to keep on dividing and replicating itself. The normal cell controls how many times it divides. An abnormal cell loses control over its own division and begins to divide randomly. This is why cancer is found in cells that normally replicate at a high rate, like skin cells, and is rarely found in cells that do not replicate rapidly like nerve cells.

Another factor is the ability of the cell to spread to another organ or different type of tissue, invade it, and keep on growing. Cells that just grow rapidly without spreading are benign tumors. For a tumor to become malignant or cancerous it needs the ability to spread.

Because cancer is a change in the cell, a sample of cells, called a biopsy, is taken. This sample is analyzed before a definite diagnosis is determined. That means that a sample of the tumor or growth must be retrieved, making the diagnosis an invasive procedure. Cancer is named by the type of cell where it starts.

Risk Factors

It is important to understand that " risk factor" is a statistical evaluation of a population. In other words, scientists looked at all the people that got a certain cancer and, after the fact, tried to make some sense of it. In order to make sense and to predict the future so they can help people detect cancer early and have a better outcome, a common link is sought. This common link is the risk factor.

So having a risk factor means an increased probability you will get the disease. But just as there are many people with the risk factor who get the disease, there are many people with the risk factor who do not get it. There are even people with no risk factors whatsoever who end up with cancer.

Your Role

You can get involved in three ways:

1. Education: In some cancers, like skin cancer and lung cancer, you can get involved in educating your clients and supporting preventative measures. Advise clients to stay out of the sun and use sunscreens and sun blocks. Encourage clients to stop smoking and to stop drinking alcohol.

2. Early detection: *Early detection is the key for survival!* The earlier a cancer is found, particularly if it is caught before it spreads in the body, the better the chance for survival and recovery. It is important to note that people with lower social economic status have higher death rates from cancer. This can be attributed to a lack of education. Once again, skin cancers are one type of cancer you can help detect for your clients. Also encourage them to have yearly check-ups.

3. *Quality of life:* Once a person is diagnosed with cancer, maintaining the quality of life becomes a major goal. The better the quality of life, the better the outcome. Read the sections on the specific cancers to learn how you can help maintain the quality of life for the cancer patient.

CHAPTER 2

Cancer Treatments

Radiation Therapy

R adiation therapy is based on the knowledge that living cells exposed to high energy will be damaged and not be able to multiply. The second fact that makes radiation therapy work is that cancerous cells multiply at a higher rate than normal cells. The result is that radiation is able to damage the rapidly multiplying cancerous cells while limiting the damage to healthy cells.

There are different types of radiation therapy. The most common one is from an outside source. The energy used is X-ray, cobalt-60 gamma ray, electron beam, neutron beam or proton beam. The beam is directed at the tumor sight on the body. The treatment is given every day for several weeks. The time of exposure is short to minimize damage to the surrounding healthy tissue. If the patient's overall health allows it, she can go home and continue with regular activities when the treatment is concluded.

Remote Brachytherapy is another type of radiation treatment which is done with an outside source of radiation that is directed through a catheter or tube directly to the tumor. This is considered an inside therapy as the beam is delivered directly into the tumor.

Another type of internal radiation is when the source of energy is implanted inside the tumor or in the area where the tumor has been removed.

A variation of this treatment is when the source is not encapsulated but the radioactive material is injected into the body. Since the radioactive material is in the body, the patient is radioactive and needs to be isolated in the hospital. Visitors and medical personnel are limited to short visits so they will not be affected by the radiation.

Side Effects of Radiation

Lack of energy is the most noticeable side effect of radiation therapy because the body is trying to heal the damaged cells. Nausea, vomiting, change of taste in the mouth and loss of appetite can also occur. Most side effects will disappear with the end of treatment.

Skin Reactions to Radiation

Skin reaction is usually delayed and can be seen two weeks or more after radiation has begun. This is because the damage that is done by radiation to the cell is only pronounced when the cell divides. The reaction can vary from red skin, swelling, itching or dry skin that is scaling. Sometimes the skin will look like it has been burned and might ulcerate. In most cases the skin will get hyper pigmented.

Some people will develop wet skin, particularly in areas were there are skin folds. Since the skin is moist, it breaks easily which increases the danger of infection.

The patient should wear pure cotton and avoid tight clothing. Itching or scratching of the irritated skin should be avoided at all costs. No heating or cooling of the sight is allowed without consulting the treating physician.

Do not apply any covering or bandages to the radiated site.

Salon Treatment of Radiation Therapy Clients

CELLS WITHOUT OXYGEN ARE NOT AFFECTED BY RADIATION. WHILE YOUR CLIENT IS GOING THROUGH RADIATION TREATMENT, DO NOT USE ANY OXYGEN TREATMENTS, OXYGEN CREAM OR OXYGEN BARS. THEY WILL INTERFERE WITH THE RADIATION TREATMENT.

IT IS IMPORTANT THAT YOU DO NOT REMOVE OR TOUCH ANY MARKINGS ON THE SKIN AS THEY ARE RADIATION GUIDES.

While undergoing radiation therapy the patient is highly advised to consult only the treating physician or nurse about skin care, including the type of soap, lotion, powder, deodorant or even sunscreen to use. The skin needs to be protected from the sun, but sunscreens can interfere with the effectiveness of the radiation. The physician needs to be consulted about the use of sunscreens.

No hair removal is allowed at the site and no depilatory lotions. If hair needs to be removed, use an electric shaver, but consult the doctor first. As for hair removal on other parts of the body consult the physician first.

It is important to know that only mild liquid cleanser and moisturizer without heavy metals should be used by the client. Remember the skin is susceptible to infections. Creams or lotions should be water based and should not contain Vaseline (petrolatum or mineral oil). If petrolatum or oil based, they can create a barrier that prevents the skin from breathing, trapping moisture and bacteria thus increasing the risk of infection. Silicones like Dimethicone are good ingredients at this stage. Vitamins, antioxidants, oxygen, peroxide, perfume, and any irritating ingredient should be avoided because they can interfere with the radiation treatment. No lotion should be applied within two hours of radiation therapy.

Salon Treatment The First Two Years After Radiation Therapy

After radiation therapy ends the use of vitamin E and silicones can be beneficial to the recovery of the skin at the site of the radiation. At this point you're treating skin that has been severely burned. Consult the physician before any treatment. Do not attempt to lighten the skin or to fight the hyper pigmentation. In time it should fade away.

Do not try to erase the radiation site markings because they might be tattoos. Avoid any aggressive treatment and any exfoliating or anti-aging treatment anywhere on the body. Recommend supportive skin care and sun screen. Clients who have undergone radiation treatments are more susceptible to skin cancer. The site of the radiation can be sensitive for a long time. Be careful when treating the skin in that area. In some patients a chronic skin reaction may occur at the sight of radiation after six to twelve months. The skin will be thin and easy to break or irritate. Scar tissue may develop under the epidermis. Permanent loss of hair at the site of treatment may occur.

Salon Treatment Two Years Or More After Radiation Therapy

If no other health conditions exist you can resume regular treatments two years after radiation treatment has ended. Radiation patients are more prone to develop skin cancer, so you need to monitor this client for any skin lesions or skin changes. Please see the Skin Cancer chapter.

Finally, as the population ages, you will be treating more and more people who have undergone radiation therapy. Now is a good time to get involved with the cancer center in your area. You might be able to work with the nurse or doctor in providing skin care to their patients.

Chemotherapy

Chemotherapy

Chemotherapy is the popular name for the treatment of cancer with drugs. This group of drugs is also called Antineoplastic agents: anti meaning against, neoplastic meaning cancer. They are also called cytotoxic: cyto meaning cell, toxic meaning poison.

The job of chemotherapy drugs is to kill cells. They are effective against cells that divide rapidly. Normal cells limit their division; cancer cells, having lost that ability, keep on multiplying and growing.

The skin and the digestive system are designed to self heal which is why their normal cells multiply at a higher rate. Even though they may be healthy they will be affected by chemotherapy. When I talk about the skin with regard to chemotherapy, I include hair and nails. When I refer to the digestive system I include the inside of the mouth and the stomach.

Chemotherapy is administered in order to eliminate the tumor, to reduce the tumor size so it can be removed by surgery or to shrink the cancer in order to reduce the tumor's effects. For example, the effect of a tumor pressing on a nerve is often pain.

Chemotherapy drugs are categorized by the mechanism of their action. The following are the traditional groups of chemotherapy drugs.

Alkylating agents which work by damaging the DNA. They are unstable molecules that bond to the DNA, damaging its structure. Once the structure is damaged, the function is damaged.

Nitrosoureas interfere with the enzymes that repair the DNA. Antimetabolites work by interfering with the normal supply of materials that are needed to build the cell, like folic acid, or by inhibiting enzymes that are critical in cell development.

Anti-tumor antibiotics interfere with the division of the cell or damage the cell membrane.

Mitotic inhibitors stop the mitotic process which is the division of the nucleus of the cell.

The next two groups are included in the pharmaceutical books under chemotherapy but are different in popular perception because of the different type of side effects.

Corticosteroids are used to slow cell growth (see page...) and are used to help with pain management as well as reduce the inflammation that can be caused by the tumor. The inflammation might be pressing on a nerve or an organ causing obstruction and pain.

Sex hormones work by blocking receptors on the tumor cells thereby eliminating the stimulation needed for the cells to divide and multiply. (see pag 36)

Chemotherapy treatment is given orally as a tablet, intravenously as an injection into the vein, by a catheter into the site of the cancer or topically with a cream or solution, as is the case with skin cancer.

The treatment is given in a series of courses where the medication is taken for a period of time, then stopped to allow the healthy cells to recuperate. Treatment can be six months or longer, depending on the cancer.

Side Effects Of Chemotherapy

Note: The side effects listed here are the ones I think you need to be aware of for your practice. There are many additional side effects that are life threatening, like damage to the liver, kidneys and lungs. Side effects have been recorded as many as 17 years after the completion of chemotherapy. The secondary cancer risk is another major problem, as any medication that cures cancer has the potential to cause cancer.

Chemotherapy is the most aggressive drug treatment known and has severe side effects. There is a delayed appearance of the side effects. Side effects will appear when the cells start dying. Tiredness or total exhaustion are common side effects because the body needs all its energy to eliminate the damaging chemicals and to heal. Nausea and vomiting will occur and can be treated with medications. Chemotherapy affects the blood system. Clotting, known as thrombocytopenia, is a common side effect. On the other end of the spectrum, excessive bleeding can also result.

Another result of chemotherapy is that veins can appear darker. It is most noticeable with darker skinned people. This will reverse itself once the drugs are eliminated from the body.

Reduction in the function of the immune system makes it easy for chemotherapy patients to become infected.

Nerve and muscle damage can appear as weakness, loss of balance, pain, tingling, burning or even numbness and loss of sensation in the hands and feet. These effects can last up to one year after chemotherapy has ended.

Depression is common. It is a reaction to the chemotherapy, the cancer itself and fear of death.

Skin Reactions

Alopecia, the loss of hair from the scalp and from the entire body including the eyebrows and eyelashes, is one of the effects women fear most. Hair will come back once chemotherapy is over. However, it might come back in a different color and or texture.

The nails can become thin and brittle with vertical lines and cracks. They may also become dark or yellow.

Skin will become sensitive, thin and will get infected easily. Skin can become dry, itchy and will be sensitive to sun. Some chemotherapy medications are phototoxic. Pre-existing conditions like acne or psoriasis may reappear.

When a patient is receiving chemotherapy the skin site of previous radiation or burn can become red and the skin can blister and peel. This can last anywhere from a few hours to several days. This reaction is called " radiation recall."

If the chemotherapy leaks or touches the skin where the IV is inserted, pain and ulceration will occur. It might require a plastic surgery correction.

Salon Treatments For Chemotherapy Clients
While on chemotherapy and up to 2 years post chemo treatment.

Before treating this client check with her treating doctor.

Patients are urged by their medical care givers to continue their normal life as part of the overall goal of maintaining a positive attitude to fight and overcome the cancer. If you choose you can get involved with your local cancer treatment center and become an integral part of the cancer support system.

Your salon or spa can become a place of refuge and provide a bit of normal routine in a crisis situation. Here are some do's and don'ts.

DO use extra precaution because these clients tend to get infected easily. Avoid any service with the potential to compromise the skin's integrity: like extraction, deep cleaning and hair removal by waxing, sugaring, threading or tweezing.

DO use only clean products and pay special attention to prevent cross contamination.

DO use a mouth mask, especially if you have been near anyone who is sick or with a cold.

DO use products that are gentle, preferably without perfumes and alcohol.

DO use moisturizing creams and lotions, the skin is dry and thin. Some beneficial ingredients are starches from oatmeal, rice or corn, silicones like Dimethicone, Aloe Vera, chamomile and zinc oxide.

DO recommend a good sun screen of at least SPF 15.

DO recommend a nail strengthener and administer a hand moisturizing treatment with warm oil. Olive oil and almond oil are beneficial.

DO help your client to get off the treatment table to prevent any falls.

DON'T peel or exfoliate the skin. Do not use chemical or botanical/ organic ingredients that thin the skin including AHA, BHA, vitamin A or C. Do not use microdermabrasion or scrubs.

DON'T use any ingredients that have the potential to be absorbed into the skin.

DON'T use any heating masks or extreme cold treatments

DON'T use body treatments like body wraps and massage of the legs because of the risk of blood clot.

DON'T suggest or recommend any oral vitamins, food supplements or any herbal remedies.

DON'T use essential oils.

Make Up

Because of hair loss, including eyebrows and lashes, your client might need your help. You can teach her how to enhance her appearance, but do not use any permanent make up. Because of the danger of infection, remind her to start with new make up and brushes. Recommend products that are water soluble, easily removed with water, containing titanium dioxide.

Salon Treatment Two Years After Chemotherapy Is Completed.

If there are no other conditions you can treat the skin as needed. Remember even after 2 years, the skin can be extremely sensitive and thin. Monitor this client for skin changes as secondary cancer may occur with chemotherapy.

Immunotherapy

Immunotherapy

Immunotherapy is a new approach in treating cancer. It is usually used in combination with another treatment like chemotherapy. Immunotherapy uses the immune system to fight cancer. There are 3 major types of immunotherapy:
1. Cancer vaccines.
2. Non-specific immune therapy which I call immune busters or immune system stimulators.
3. Monoclonal Antibody therapy (MAbs).

Cancer Vaccine

Cancer vaccines are being investigated for all major cancers and are currently available only through clinical trials. There are 2 kinds of cancer vaccines: Autologous vaccines, extracted from the patient, and Allogenic vaccines, developed from other patients.

The vaccines include cancer cells, parts of cells or antigens. The theory is that the body will react to the foreign material and the immune system will then fight not only the new material but also the cancer cells in the body. The reaction is thought to be specific to the cancer itself. Since this is a new approach there is currently no full information on side effects and contraindications.

Immune busters

The theory behind immune busters is that if the body has more of the substance that initiates the body's immune response then the immune system reaction is going to be stronger, and the body will have more protecting, fighting and correcting ability. The body's immune system is awakened when the body is invaded by foreign intruders like viruses and bacteria. One reaction for example, is the development of a fever when you get a cold. These drugs are used in combination with other cancer treatments like chemotherapy and radiation. This type of treatment is new and most of the drugs are still investigational which means they are only used experimentally and are not available to all patients.

This field is still evolving, and new components of the immune system are being discovered. The two groups of drugs currently available are the Interferons and the Interleukins

Interferons

Interferons are proteins or glycoproteins that are produced by cells when the cells are being attacked. In simple terms, interferons are the "message" being sent for the body to boost its immune system.

They are being used in cancer treatment to stimulate the body's immune response so the body can fight the cancer. They are used also to treat viral infections like HIV and hepatitis.

There are 3 types of Interferons: Interferon alpha, Interferon beta and Interferon gamma. In each type there are sub-types. Interferons can be produced by genetic engineering, or they can be extracted from human or animal living cells.

Since they are proteins they need to be given by injection under the skin, or into the muscle. They can also be injected directly into the blood intravenously.

The treatment is usually one injection daily for up to 6 months.

Side Effects

The most common side effect is flu like symptoms. The patient is weak, and a fever may be present. Interferons can aggravate pre-existing conditions like psoriasis.

Salon treatment

In general a client who is going through treatment with interferons is in grave condition. After consulting with the treating physician, you can give a basic European facial using only the mildest ingredients.

Interferons interfere with the liver's capability to clear medications out of the body, therefore you should avoid using any skin care that is absorbed into the body including aromatherapy and vitamin A. Blood clots can occur, so massage therapy and body wraps should be avoided. Six month following final treatment and if there are no other contraindications, (remember this patient might have also gotten chemotherapy, or radiation or both) you can treat the skin per the skin's needs.

Interleukins

Interleukin is a cell produced protein that is involved in the hormonal regulation of the immune response. It is a relatively new group that is being investigated in treating cancer. Interleukins are used with chemotherapy and radiation to boost the immune system. Some of the Interleukins available are: Interluken 1 alpha and 1 beta, Interleukin 2, Interleukin 3,4,5,7,8 and Interleukin 6 which is used with breast cancer patients.

Interleukins are produced through genetic engineering or by extraction from living cells.

Side Effects

They all produce flu like symptoms, but all possible side effects are currently unknown.

Monoclonal Antibody therapy (MAbs)

Since the immune system is not being stimulated MAbs is considered to be a passive therapy. MAbs are laboratory produced antibodies that work even when the immune system is weakened. They are specific antibodies that react with a specific antigen on the cancer cell. They can be naked or loaded.

Naked MAbs work by themselves. They connect to the cancer

cell either to block a specific molecule binding site, or they become a marker for the immune system so that it recognizes the cancer cell as an enemy and fights the cancer.

Loaded MAbs (conjugated, tagged, labeled, chemolabeled) carry chemotherapy drugs, radioactive materials or toxins to the cancer cell. The MAbs act as a "guide" bringing the drugs directly where they are needed to maximize the effect. The hope is that in the future this sophisticated method will minimize the dangerous effect on the healthy cells and reduce the side effects thus making cancer-fighting treatment more comfortable. At this time MAbs are looking very promising, but most are still only available as investigational drugs.

Severe side effects have been reported including allergic reactions and heart problems. MAbs have only been in use for a year, and it will take time until we know about their effects on the skin.

New anticancer therapies are being developed all over the world. I encourage you to follow up by consulting the reference list at the end of the book for the exciting new approaches to cancer therapy.

Bone Marrow Transplantation

Bone Marrow Transplantation

B one marrow transplant is a generic term that includes the harvesting of different stem cells and transplanting them. The stem cells that produce blood and immune cells are located in the bone marrow. This procedure increases the quantity of the desired stem cells, and as a result, a larger number of healthy cells will be produced.

A bone marrow transplant is done when the stem cells are malignant or when there are not enough stem cells because they have been killed with high doses of radiation or chemotherapy. Bone marrow can be frozen and thawed making this procedure readily available. Once marrow is located it is aspirated from the posterior or anterior iliac crest. It is cleaned and processed then infused into the chest bone.

There are two sources of bone marrow. Bone marrow can be obtained from the patient's own marrow, which is called autologous. Bone marrow can be taken from another person, a donor. This is referred to as allogenic. The donor can be a family member or not.

The probability that a non-family member will be a match is only about 1 in 10,000. In the US there is a National Marrow Donor Program with more then 3 million volunteers. It takes three to four months to find a match. Today, about half of all transplant patients find a match through this program. The chances of finding a match with a family member are better than 50%.

Side Effects

The problem with a bone marrow transplant is rejection. When the marrow transplant uses the patient's own bone marrow there is no problem. If the patient is lucky enough to have an identical twin there will also be no problem with rejection. But with a family member or an unrelated donor, there can be a rejection. To overcome the possibility of rejection, the patient is given medications, like corticosteroids, that shut down the immune system. This makes the patient susceptible to infections.

The first 3 months after the transplant are critical, but some patients require medication for up to three years after the transplant. Because of the risk of infections, antibiotics and antiviral medications are also prescribed. The first sign of a problem will be the appearance of a rash.

Salon Treatment

Before treating a client who has had a bone marrow transplant consult the treating doctor. If the client has taken steroids in the two year period after the treatment ends, the skin will be thin, slow to heal and susceptible to infection.

DON'T use any skin thinning treatments including hair removal, microdermabrasion or anti-aging treatments.

DO use skin care treatment that is gentle and supportive to the skin.

DO encourage your client to wear sun screen.

After two years

You can resume regular skin treatments two years after the end of all medical treatments related to the bone marrow transplant if no other medical conditions exist.

Corticosteroids

Corticosteroids
Prednisone

Prednisone, a corticosteroid, is a potent drug. It is prescribed for cancer patients to reduce swelling, tumor size and to prevent rejection of the bone marrow transplant.

Depending on the condition, a patient can take it for a week or for years, as is the case with bone marrow transplants.

As with any potent drug, Prednisone has many side effects. Three affect the skin directly; skin thinning, healing time reduction and infection masking.

Skin Thinning

Dermal atrophy(thinning of the skin) makes the need for exfoliating services or ingredients absolutely unnecessary. The skin is already thin because of the medication, and it heals slowly. You need to avoid: AHA, BHA, Vitamin A and Vitamin C in high concentrations. It also makes waxing hair removal unsafe for a period of 6 months from the time Prednisone treatment ended.

Infection Masking

Masking of infections occurs because Prednisone reduces the inflammation, redness and itchiness associated with the infection process. Although you may not see clear symptoms, the infection is still evolving.

Because of the increased sensitivity to infections and the effect of masking, it is a good idea to use extra precaution. Make sure your equipment and products are clean so you will not cause infection.

If your client suffers from acne, psoriasis or rosacea you may see a flare up while she is being treated with Prednisone or when she gets off the medication. You may also see steroidal acne (it can be diagnosed by the dermatologist). Conventional salon treatments or cosmetic ingredients can reduce the redness or irritation, but this problem will not go away until the medication is stopped.

Other Side effects

It is unfortunate that women who take Prednisone for a long period of time will develop dark course facial hair, similar to a man's. On the other hand, they may experience Alopecia (loss of hair on the head).

Because of potential increased blood pressure and fluid retention you should avoid salon treatments that stimulate blood flow to the heart.

Salon treatments for clients who are taking Prednisone
(This applies for six months following cessation of medication.)

DON'T exfoliate

DON'T use AHAs, BHAs, Vitamin A, Vitamin C serums

DON'T remove hair by waxing until 6 months after prednisone medication has ceased.

DON'T use treatments that increase blood flow to the heart.

Hormonal Therapy

Hormonal Therapy

Tamoxifen

Tamoxifen, sold under the brand name Nolvadex, is a drug being prescribed to prevent breast cancer. Tamoxifen is an antiestrogen drug usually prescribed following surgery for breast cancer. It is used in conjunction with chemotherapy or radiation. A five-year study indicates that women who took Tamoxifen were forty-five percent less likely to develop cancer than women who did not. However, the study also indicated that there are two known side effects of Tamoxifen —uterine cancer and blood clots.

When a client suffers from blood clots, you should avoid body wraps or massage to the lower extremities because these treatments increase the risk of blood clots that can travel to the heart and lungs possibly creating a life-threatening situation. Note: Massage therapy can be beneficial in preventing blood clots.

In some women nausea and vomiting can be induced by fragrances, pressure to the chest, and or pressure to the abdominal area. Women taking Tamoxifen also experience a higher rate of hot flashes. Edema, skin rashes and dry skin can also result. If the client suffers from dry skin be sure and use appropriate creams. Dizziness, headaches, depression, confusion, fatigue and muscle cramps have also been reported by users of Tamoxifin.

Salon treatment for clients taking Tamoxifen

DON'T use body warps or massage on lower extremities.
DON'T use pressure on chest or abdomen
DON'T use strong fragrances.
DO use moisturizing and protecting products
DO recommend sunscreen
DO support the skin with salon treatments and products.

CALL THE TREATING PHYSICIAN BEFORE YOU ADMINISTER ANY SALON TREATMENT TO A CANCER PATIENT, A RECOVERING CANCER PATIENT OR A FORMER CANCER PATIENT.

CHAPTER 3

Skin Cancer

Skin Cancer

I will open with a personal note to the skin care professional. I ask you to please pay close attention to this chapter. This chapter talks about cancer of the skin, the organ you see, touch and treat. This is the one cancer that you can help detect and prevent. This is one more place where I see you as a crucial and essential part of your client's well being. Not only can you help prevent this disease but you can also help with early detection, possibly prolonging life and minimizing suffering.

Although you will get a good understanding of skin cancer from this chapter, I urge you to absorb as much information as you can about this disease.

Please use the reference list in the end of the book. Please keep in mind the saying that it is better to be safe than sorry. Do not be afraid to ask questions and to refer your client to a dermatologist if you have even the slightest suspicion.

When one hears the word skin cancer it is clear that the cancer is on the skin, but it really is not telling you any more than that. It is almost like saying this is a child but you do not know any more details; like how tall the child is, how old the child is, or even if it is a boy or a girl.

The names of skin cancers are designated by the type of the cell where the cancer starts to grow.

Skin cancer is divided into two groups: Melanoma and Nonmelanoma. Nonmelanoma is further divided into different subgroups. Nonmelanoma also includes the pre-cancerous condition Actinic Keratosis. The first question to ask is, " Is it Melanoma or Nonmelanoma?"

Nonmelanoma skin cancers (NMSC)

Nonmelanoma skin cancers (NMSC) are the most common cancers in the US. There are more than 1 million new cases diagnosed every year. NMSC includes cancerous and pre-cancerous conditions. The two most common cancerous NMSC are Basal Cell Carcinoma (BCC), making up 70 to 80% and Squamos Cell Carcinoma, making up the other 20% of all cases. Although not a cancer Actinic Keratosis is included in this chapter because it is a common precancerous condition that may evolve into Squamos Cell Carcinoma.

Risk factors for NMSC

There is no doubt that the main reason and cause of NMSC is exposure to the sun, in particular Ultraviolet B spectrum (UVB) light.

NMSC is most common on the face, neck and ears. Men have more cases than women. If you doubt that exposure to the sun is linked directly to cancer consider this fact. In England more cases of NCMS occur on the right side of the face because the English drive on the left side of the road. Here in the U.S., where we drive on the right hand side of the road, there are more occurrences on the left side of the face.

People that live in colder climates, farther away from the equator, like Minneapolis or Chicago, have less incidence of NMSC than people who live in warmer, sun loving cities like Miami and Los Angeles.

NMSC is more prevalent in fair skinned populations. So a fair skinned person who is easily sun burned is more likely to develop NMSC than a person with darker skin.

Based on that, you can see why sun beds should not be used at all. As a skin care professional, you need to teach your clients to avoid sun bathing and sun tanning in nature or with artificial sources.

The workplace can be a factor. What a person does for a living will give you one more source of information to see if they are at risk for developing NMSC. Outdoor occupations where your client spends most of the day exposed to the UVB rays (290-320 nm) is one such group. The other group is people who are exposed to heat, like people who work in restaurants next to hot oils. Extended exposure to heat will create the same damaging inflammation process of the skin that can result in NMSC.

Age is also a risk factor. As a person gets older, the more likely they are to develop cancer. Clients over the age of 40 are the ones to be especially concerned with. Other risk factors for NMSC include:

1. Chronic trauma, like wounds, ulcers and scars.
2. Cigarette smoking, which will increase lip and oral cancer.
3. Exposure to arsenic through water or food.
4. Tar in topical application, in particular the cyclic aromatic hydrocarbons in the tar.
5. Viral infection (human papilloma virus).
6. Radiation treatment.
7. Genetics, particularly people of Celtic descent.

Basal Cell Carcinoma (BCC)

Description & Detection

The problem with BCC is that it is very hard to detect because it resembles other common skin conditions— eczema , psoriasis or a small wound. The other problem is that it may look small outside, while it spreads unnoticed on the inside.

If BCC is not treated it destroys the tissue surrounding it. It can destroy the face on the outside while spreading into the bone and the brain on the inside. The good news with BBC is that it grows slowly. It stays localized and does not spread through the blood or the lymph system. The other very good news is that if it is discovered early, it can be treated successfully.

You need to look for wounds on your client that return in the same place. If it bleeds or scales with or without pain, this is a warning sign — refer your client to a dermatologist immediately. Twenty-five to thirty percent of BCC will occur on the nose. It can also develop on the face, neck, scalp or ears. It rarely occurs on the back of the hands or on the trunk of the body.

Although BCC is not considered to be a life threatening cancer; if not treated, it can be devastating and even life altering.

BCC Types

Nodular BCC

There are several types of BCC, the most common being Nodular BCC. As its name implies, it looks like a little nodule or raised bump. It has a pearly color and a smooth or pebbly surface. As it grows you might see dialated blood vessels through the thin skin. You might even mistakenly think it is a milia. As it extends it might break, bleed or create an ulcer. Once the ulceration occurs, it has a new name, Nodulo-ulcerative BCC. The ulcer heals as it crusts and scales. That is when it might be thought of as " not a problem". But the lesion keeps growing and expanding on the inside. This dangerous cycle continues.

Superficial Spreading BCC

Superficial spreading BCC is thin, almost flat wound that looks like the fungal infection "tinea corporis". It is most common on the trunk of the body. It scales and grows horizontally and slowly.

Morpheaform BCC

Morpheaform BCC looks like a scar or regular skin, and it grows mostly inwards. It can be pigmented and therefore look like melanoma.

Pinkus Tumor BCC

Pinkus tumor is more easily detected. It looks like a large skin tag and grows on the trunk of older men.

Medical Treatments for BCC

The treatment of BCC depends on the site and size of the tumor, the age of the patient and other medical considerations. The goal is to get rid of all the cancerous cells. This is achieved by scraping the tumor (curettage) then stopping the bleeding with an electrical probe (electrodessication).

Other methods of removal include freezing with liquid nitrogen (cryosurgery), burning with radiation or laser. When the tumor is larger it is removed by a cutting procedure called Moh's micrographic surgery. Patients may experience pain, crusting and oozing up to 6 weeks after the procedure. You will be interested to know that it takes one to two years of special training for a dermatologist to be qualified to do Moh's surgery.

Most patients treated will be cured. But keep in mind that patients that have had one type of skin cancer are more likely to develop other skin cancers.

BCC Salon Treatments

Before considering any treatment please contact the treating physician. Please do not recommend any skin care product, essential oils or herbal remedies for either external or internal use until the wound has completely healed.

Based on the facts about skin cancer, a frightening connection surfaces. Salon treatment and cosmetic products that constantly thin the skin, therefore making it more sensitive to sun exposure, and those treatments and products that traumatize the skin by chemical burning, pressure or abrasion have the potential to promote cancer growth in the very clients you are trying to help, namely, fair skinned clients with the more noticeable sun damage and age spots. A better solution is to advocate sun prevention practice.

Squamous Cell Carcinoma (SCC)

Description & Detection

SCC is a skin cancer that has the potential to spread to other organs and become fatal. The lesion is measured by depth. Any lesion thicker than 4 millimeters can be life threatening. Any lesion thicker than 10 millimeters is considered fatal.

SCC can develop on sun-exposed areas of the body: the scalp, back of hands, lips, ears, face, neck. It can also appear anywhere else on the body.

SCC develops in middle-aged adults. You can expect to see more cases as clients age. Men are twice as likely to get SCC as women. SCC develops in the epithelium where the repair system of the cell has been damaged. Scientists have been able to identify the gene in charge of repairing damage done during the cell's development, thereby preventing irregular abnormal cells from growing. They have given that tumor suppression gene the identifying number p53.

The lesion can look like a BCC, actinic keratosis or a wart. Most of the time it will initially look like a red lesion with rough texture and no clear borders. It can be raised and dark like a bloody wound crust that can scale and bleed, or it can look like a swollen-bordered deep ulcer that does not heal. The lesion can grow rapidly and can spread undetected under the surface of the skin.

Risk Factors for SCC

UV damage from the sun plays a major role in this life threatening disease.

Other common factors are actinic keratosis, chronic infection, burn scars, radiation exposure and chemical exposure to non therapeutic tar and arsenic.

UVB radiation damages the p53 gene, thus eliminating the cell's ability to repair. In addition, a weak immune system will allow SCC to develop more quickly. For example, patients whose immune system is weakened are 253 times more likely to get SCC than the normal population. SCC will proliferate in the body via the lymphatic system.

Medical Treatment for SCC

Treatment varies by factors like the size and site of the SCC and the age of the patient. Small SCC are removed like BCC. SCC larger than 4 mm are removed and the surrounding area is treated with radiation and chemotherapy.

Radiation therapy is based on the knowledge that living cells exposed to high energy will be damaged and not be able to multiply. The second fact that makes radiation therapy work is that cancerous cells multiply at a higher rate then normal cells. The result is that radiation is able to damage the rapidly multiplying cancerous cells while limiting the damage to healthy cells.

There are different types of radiation therapy. The most common one is from an outside source. The energy used is X-ray, cobalt-60 gamma ray, electron beam, neutron beam or proton beam. The beam is directed at the tumor sight on the body. The treatment is given every day for several weeks. The time of the exposure is short to minimize damage to the surrounding healthy tissue. If the patient's overall health allows it, she can go home and continue with regular activities when the treatment is concluded.

Side Effects of Radiation

Lack of energy is the most noticeable side effect of radiation therapy because the body is trying to heal the damaged cells. Nausea, vomiting, change of taste in the mouth and loss of appetite can also occur. Most side effects will disappear with the end of treatment.

Skin Reactions to Radiation

Skin reaction is usually delayed and can usually be seen after two weeks or more after radiation has begun because the damage that is done by radiation to the cell is only pronounced when the cell divides. The reaction can vary from red skin, swelling, itching or dry skin that is scaling. Sometimes the skin will look like it has been burned and might ulcerate. In most cases the skin will get hyper pigmented.

Some people will develop wet skin, particularly in areas were there are skin folds. Since the skin is moist, it breaks easily which increases the danger of infection.

The patient should wear pure cotton and avoid tight clothing. Itching or scratching of the irritated skin should be avoided at all costs. No heating or cooling of the sight is allowed without consulting the treating physician. Do not apply any covering or bandages to the radiated site.

Salon Treatment of Squamos Cell Carcinoma (SCC)

PLEASE REMEMBER THAT LYMPHATIC DRAINAGE TREATMENTS CAN ACCELERATE THE SPREAD OF SCC IN THE BODY.

Salon treatment of SCC radiation therapy client

While undergoing radiation therapy the patient is highly advised to consult only the treating physician or nurse about skin care, including the type of soap, lotion, powder, deodorant or even sunscreen to use. The skin needs to be protected from the sun, but sunscreens can interfere with the effectiveness of the radiation. The physician needs to be consulted about the use of sunscreens.

No hair removal or depilatory lotions are allowed at the site. If hair needs to be removed, use an electric shaver, but consult the doctor first. As for hair removal on other parts of the body, consult the physician first.

It is important that only mild liquid cleansers and moisturizers that do not contain heavy metals should be used by the client. Remember, the skin is susceptible to infections. Creams or lotions should be water based and should not contain Vaseline (petrolatum or mineral oil). If petrolatum or oil based, they can create a barrier that prevents the skin from breathing, thus trapping moisture and bacteria and increasing the risk of infection. Silicones like Dimethicone are good ingredients at this stage. Vitamins, antioxidants, oxygen, peroxide, perfume and any irritating ingredient should be avoided because they can interfere with the radiation treatment. No lotion should be applied within two hours of radiation therapy.

Salon Treatment The First Two Years After Radiation Therapy

After radiation therapy ends the use of vitamin E and silicones can be beneficial to the recovery of the skin at the radiation site. At this point you have skin that has been severely burned. Consult the physician before any treatment. Do not attempt to lighten the skin or to fight the hyper pigmentation. In time it should fade away.

Do not try to erase the radiation site markings because they might be tattoos. Avoid any aggressive treatment and any exfoliating or anti-aging treatment anywhere on the body.

Recommend supportive skin care and sunscreen. Clients who have undergone radiation treatments are more susceptible to skin cancer. The site of the radiation can be sensitive for a long time. Be careful when treating the skin in that area. In some patients a chronic skin reaction will occur at the site of radiation after six to twelve months. The skin will be thin and easily break, or irritate. Scar tissue may develop under the epidermis. Permanent loss of hair at the site of treatment may occur.

Salon Treatment Two Or More Years After Radiation Therapy

If no other health conditions exist you can resume regular treatments two years after the radiation treatment has ended. Radiation patients are more prone to develop skin cancers, so you need to monitor this client for any skin lesions or skin changes.

Finally, as the population and your clients age, you will treat more and more people who have undergone radiation therapy. Now is a good time to get involved with the cancer center in your area. You might be able to work with the nurse or doctor in providing better, safer skin care to their patients.

ALWAYS RECOMMEND SUN SCREENS

For salon treatments for the chemotherapy patient (see page 63)

Precancerous Skin Lesions
Actinic Keratosis

IT IS IMPORTANT TO BE AWARE OF THIS SKIN CONDITION AS IT CAN TURN INTO SQUAMOS CELL CARCINOMA.

Description & Detection

Actinic Keratosis is the most common precancerous condition. It can turn into Squamos Cell Carcinoma.

Actinic Keratosis develops in sun-damaged skin, typically in the areas of the forehead, scalp, ears, neck, shoulders, face and the back of the hands. It can also develop in other areas. It takes many years of growth until lesions become visible. Actinic Keratosis is common in mature, light skinned people who have been extensively exposed to the sun. The cells involved are Squamous cells in the epidermis which become abnormal or atypical. The change in these cells, which can be seen in a microscope, causes the cells to function in a way that is different from a normal cell. The manifestation seen with the naked eye is irregular skin with a rough texture bump. This evolves into a persistent red wound that later develops a yellow crust that thickens. When this scab falls off, the wound bleeds, and new crust will be created. It can start as a single wound or a few spots and involve the entire forehead or scalp.

There is a slight possibility that the lesions will go into remission and disappear, but that does not mean the lesions will not come back. At a very slow rate Actinic Keratosis cells progress and transform into SCC cells. The estimate is that only 2 to 5 % make this transformation, but we know that 60% of all SCC started as actinic keratosis. This is why this skin condition is included in this chapter and why you need to be familiar with it.

Risk Factors

See NMSC section page 45 for risk factors.

Actinic Cheilitis

Description & Detection

Actinic Cheilitis is the name given to the more aggressive form of Actinic Keratosis of the lower border of the lip vermilion. If it goes undetected it can progress into SCC. SCC which develops from actinic cheilitis is one of the most aggressive, fastest growing and life threatening cancers.

If your client has a persistent dryness of the lips please refer her to the doctor because this can be a sign of Actinic Cheilitis. (See Risk Factors and Medical Treatment section under Medical Treatments for BCC)

Medical Treatment Actinic Keratosis & Actinic Cheilitis

The goal of the treatment is to kill all the cells that are atypical and thereby prevent the possibility that those abnormal cells will become cancer cells.

When the number of lesions is small, most physicians will choose to eliminate the cells by freezing with liquid nitrogen. This is known as Cryotherapy and is the most effective method. After freezing, the patient might experience a burn like pain, but it is the quickest and the safest treatment. Cryotherapy can cause hypopigmentation or white spots to appear on the skin of darker skinned people. For this reason it is not used on large areas for darker skinned patients.

If the crust is thick the physicians might remove it with surgery or laser.

Topical chemotherapy

Larger areas are treated with 5-FU (5-fluorouracil). This is a topical antineoplastic medication in the form of a cream. It is manufactured in different strengths. Carac, the brand name manufactured by Dermik, comes in a 0.5% solution. Efudex manufactured by ICN comes in a 5% cream and in 2% and 5 % solutions.Efudex solution is usually prescribed for application on the scalp.

The cream or the solution will be applied either several times daily or in some cases, once a week. The patient will experience a fair amount of discomfort. The medication prevents the atypical cells from growing, and the skin will become inflamed, causing pain. The wounds will become ulcerated and then heal. The treatment takes three to eight weeks, depending on the inflammation and the patient.

Actinex (masoprocol) is another topical medication. Patients find it is more tolerable than 5-FU, but it is not as effective.

Retin A is used in early stages, but if the wound does not respond within two to four months, then a more aggressive treatment is used.

Chemical peels, Glycolic acid, TCA, or Jessner's Solution are used topically on the lesions, alone or in combination with 5-FU treatment.

After treatment, most lesions are expected to be eliminated for months or even years, but they can return. It is crucial that you do not attempt to treat any new lesions in the salon. It is as important to encourage the client to see the doctor as soon as possible.

Salon Treatment of Actinic Keratosis

DANGER: DO NOT TREAT ACTINIC KERATOSIS IN THE SALON BECAUSE THE SURFACE MIGHT LOOK HEALED BUT PRECANCEROUS CELLS MAY REMAIN HIDDEN UNDER THE SURFACE AND KEEP ON GROWING.

First and foremost I see you as a very important part of the detection process. You are the one who sees and touches the skin. You are the one with the trained eye who can recognize when the skin does not look normal. If you have even the slightest suspicion that there is something abnormal about your client's skin, please refer them to the doctor.

Second, you play a crucial part in prevention. Educate your clients to stay out of the sun and teach them the proper use of sunscreens. Do not forget to recommend and sell proper sunscreens in the salon. Follow up and remind your client to keep plenty of sunscreen on hand and purchase a new tube before she runs out.

Third, once your client is diagnosed with actinic keratosis and is undergoing treatment, you can help by consulting with the doctor, and then suggesting a gentle skin cleanser and a gentle moisturizer. The skin needs to be clean and dry before application of 5-FU. A moisturizer and a sunscreen can be applied two hours after the application of 5-FU. Please make sure these products do not contain any AHA or BHA, vitamin C or vitamin A as these ingredients can interfere with treatment. If the treatment is 5-FU, these ingredients can induce pain and will change the absorption rate and efficacy of the medication.

Fourth, after the completion of therapy, hyperpigmentation may be extensive. Do not use any bleaching or skin lightening product on the client.

Fifth, when the skin heals - moisturizing, nourishing and European facials can be of great benefit. It is my opinion that it is important for the client to see you on a regular basis, every four to six weeks. Their skin will need your help. Gentle facials in the salon, and proper products for home use will help the recovery process. Ingredients like vitamin E and dimethicone will help protect the skin from the environment and support the proper functioning of the skin.

Any exfoliating ingredient like AHA or BHA, any vitamin A, vitamin C or any microdermabrasion should be avoided because they will further "thin" the skin and expose it to the damaging sun. They can also mask atypical cell growth and prevent early detection.

Lymphatic drainage should not be done because you might mobilize cancerous cells and expedite their spread throughout the body.

Melanoma

IT IS IMPORTANT FOR EVERY ONE TO PAY ATTENTION. LEARN WHAT TO LOOK FOR. YOU CAN SAVE A WOMAN'S LIFE.

Melanoma is known as the aggressive skin cancer that kills. It develops in the melanocite, the cell that is responsible for producing the color of the skin. That is the reason that melanoma is manifested as a pigmented tumor. When it spreads, it travels via the lymphatic system or the blood system and can consequently invade other organs like the liver, lungs, brain and bones. There are 44,200 new cases every year. There are 7,300 deaths every year from Melanoma. The good news is that it is easy to detect and, if detected early, can be stopped and cured before it spreads.

GET TO KNOW WHAT MELANOMA LOOKS LIKE. YOU CAN SAVE A LIFE.

What does Melanoma look like?

Here's an easy way to identify a Melanoma. It's called the A-B-C- D characteristics. If you can remember your ABC's, it easy to identify a Melanoma:

     A. Asymmetry

     B. Borders

     C. Color

     D. Diameter

Asymmetry When one looks at the lesion it looks irregular in shape. It does not look like a circle or an oval. For example, if you could fold the lesion in half, one side would not be equal to the other.

Borders There is no clear border. It looks like the normal skin is mixed with the lesion, and there is no clear line between the two.

Color Melanoma lesions always have color because they are developing in a melanocite cell that is growing out of control. This out of control cell is producing the color in the skin. Because it is growing irregularly, the lesion has a dark color that is not unified. There are areas with lighter and darker colors. Color can vary from brown to black to blue, white and red. In comparison a normal mole will have one color, usually brown. If there is a variation, it will be equally distributed over the entire area of the mole.

Diameter Most melanomas are larger than 6mm, but there have been smaller lesions that were malignant. Bleeding occurs late in the evolvement of the melanoma and at this point the prognosis is bleak. The bad news is that it can appear even in young people, and it is extremely dangerous. The other bad news is more and more people are expected to have melanoma. By the year 2010 one out of every 100 people, or 1% of the population is expected to have melanoma.

MELANOMA CAN APPEAR ANYWHERE ON THE BODY. IT IS IMPORTANT TO PAY ATTENTION TO AREAS THAT ARE NORMALLY HIDDEN FROM VIEW.

Types of Melanoma
Superficial Spreading Malignant Melanoma (SSMM)
The most common type is Superficial Spreading Malignant Melanoma (SSMM). It appears between the ages of forty to fifty and can occur on any part of the body. It is most common on the back for men and on the back and on the legs below the knees on women.

Lentigo Malignant Melanoma (LMM)

This is common in people who are sixty to seventy years old and appears areas of the body exposed to the sun. 90% of LMM occurs on the face. The other 10% of the cases appear on other exposed areas, like the arms.

Arcal lentiginous melanoma (ALM)

Another type is Arcal lentiginous melanoma (ALM). Most patients that get ALM are African Americans or Asians. It appears most commonly on the palms of the hands, the soles of the feet and on the proximal nail fold.

Be aware Melanoma can develop on any part of the skin, including between the toes, under the nail bed and in the rectal and vaginal areas.

Risk Factors for Melanoma

Most cases of Melanoma occur in light or freckle skinned people with blonde or red hair and blue or light eyes. People who sunburn easily are also at risk. People who have lived in sunny places like California, Florida, Israel or Australia before they were 10 years old are also at risk. Melanoma is rare in darker skinned people, but it also occurs in these populations.

Here again exposure to the sun, particularly at a young age, is the biggest risk factor.

Genetics also plays a significant role. One out of every 10 people with this cancer, will have a family member with the disease. In medical terms, this is considered a family history.

Another risk factor is a mole, known medically as a nevi. All moles have the potential to become cancerous. The risk of a regular mole becoming cancerous is minimal. Atypical moles and large congenital moles like birthmarks have a high risk of becoming malignant. It might be a good idea to ask a physician to remove this type of mole.

Medical Treatment of Melanoma:

Treatment depends on the stage of the melanoma. If discovered early surgical removal will be the most efficacious treatment. Removal of the lymph nodes closest to the tumor are usually part of the procedure.

If the melanoma has spread, or is suspected to have spread, then chemotherapy will be administered.

Chemotherapy is the popular name for the treatment of cancer with drugs. This group of drugs is also called Antineoplastic agents: anti meaning against, neoplastic meaning cancer. They are also called Cytotoxic: cyto meaning cell, toxic meaning poison.

The job of chemotherapy drugs is to kill cells. They are effective against cells that divide rapidly. Normal cells limit their division; cancer cells, having lost that ability, keep on multiplying and growing.

The skin and the digestive system are designed to self heal which is why their normal cells multiply at a higher rate. Even though they may be healthy they will be affected by chemotherapy. When I talk about the skin with regard to chemotherapy, I include hair and nails. When I refer to the digestive system I include the inside of the mouth and the stomach.

Chemotherapy is administered in order to eliminate the tumor, to reduce the tumor size so it can be removed by surgery or to shrink the cancer in order to reduce the tumor's effects. For example, the effect of a tumor pressing on a nerve is often pain

Chemotherapy treatment is given orally as a tablet, intravenously as an injection into the vein, or by a catheter into the site of the cancer.

The treatment is given in a series of courses where the medication is taken for a period of time, then stopped to allow the healthy cells to recuperate. Treatment can be six months or longer, depending on the cancer.

Side Effects Of Chemotherapy

Note: The side effects listed here are the ones I think you need to be aware of for your practice. There are many additional side effects that are life threatening, like damage to the liver, kidneys and lungs. Side effects have been recorded as many as 17 years after the completion of chemotherapy. The secondary cancer risk is another major problem, as any medication that cures cancer has the potential to cause cancer.

Chemotherapy is the most aggressive drug treatment known and has severe side effects. There is a delayed appearance of the side effects. Side effects will appear when the cells start dying. Tiredness or total exhaustion are common side effects because the body needs all its energy to eliminate the damaging chemicals and to heal. Nausea and vomiting will occur and can be treated with medications.

Chemotherapy affects the blood system. Clotting, known as thrombocytopenia, is a common side effect. On the other end of the spectrum, excessive bleeding can also result.

Another result of chemotherapy is that veins can appear darker. It is most noticeable with darker skinned people. This will reverse itself once the drugs are eliminated from the body.

Reduction in the function of the immune system makes it easy for chemotherapy patients to become infected.

Nerve and muscle damage can appear as weakness, loss of balance, pain, tingling, burning or even numbness and loss of sensation in the hands and feet. These effects can last up to one year after chemotherapy has ended.

Depression is common. It is a reaction to the chemotherapy, the cancer itself and fear of death.

Skin Reactions

Alopecia, the loss of hair from the scalp and from the entire body including the eyebrows and eyelashes, is one of the effects women fear most. Hair will come back once chemotherapy is over. However, it might come back in a different color and or texture.

The nails can become thin and brittle with vertical lines and cracks. They may also become dark or yellow.

Skin will become sensitive, thin and will get infected easily. Skin can become dry, itchy and will be sensitive to sun. Some chemotherapy medications are phototoxic. Preexisting conditions like acne or psoriasis may reappear.

When a patient is receiving chemotherapy the skin site of previous radiation or burn can become red and the skin can blister and peel. This can last anywhere from a few hours to several days. This reaction is called " Radiation recall."

If the chemotherapy leaks or touches the skin where the IV is inserted, pain and ulceration will occur. It might require a plastic surgery correction.

Salon Treatment of Melanoma

Salon Treatments For Chemotherapy Clients
While on chemotherapy and for 2 years post chemo-treatment.

Before treating this client check with her treating doctor.

Patients are urged by their medical care givers to continue their normal life as part of the overall goal of maintaining a positive attitude to fight and overcome the cancer.

If you choose you can get involved with your local cancer treatment center and become an integral part of the cancer support system.

Your salon or spa can become a place of refuge and provide a bit of normal routine in a crisis situation. Here are some do's and don'ts.

DO use extra precaution because these clients tend to get infected easily. Avoid any service with the potential to compromise the skin's integrity: like extraction, deep cleaning, hair removal by waxing, sugaring, threading or tweezing.

DO use only clean products and pay special attention to prevent cross contamination.

DO use a mouth mask, especially if you have been near anyone who is sick or with a cold.

DO use products that are gentle, preferably without perfumes and alcohol.

DO use moisturizing creams and lotions, the skin is dry and thin. Some beneficial ingredients are starches from oatmeal, rice and corn, silicones like Dimethicone, Aloe Vera, chamomile and zinc oxide.

DO recommend a good sun screen of at least SPF 15.

DO recommend a nail strengthener and administer a hand moisturizing treatment with warm oil. Olive oil and almond oil are beneficial.

DO help your client to get off the treatment table to prevent any falls.

DON'T peel or exfoliate the skin. Do not use chemical or botanical/organic ingredients that thin the skin including AHA, BHA, vitamin A or C. Do not use microdermabrasion or scrubs.

DON'T use any ingredients that have the potential to be absorbed into the skin.

DON'T use any heating masks or extreme cold treatments

DON'T use body treatments like body wraps and massage of the legs because of the risk of blood clot.

DON'T suggest or recommend any oral vitamins, food supplements
or any herbal remedies
DON'T use essential oils.

Make Up

Because of hair loss, including eyebrows and lashes, your client might need your help. You can teach her how to enhance her appearance, but do not use any permanent make up. Because of the danger of infection, remind her to start with new make up and brushes. Recommend products that are water soluble, that are easily removed with water, containing titanium dioxide.

Salon Treatment Two Years After Chemotherapy Is Completed

If there are no other conditions you can treat the skin as needed. Remember even after 2 years, the skin can be extremely sensitive and thin. Monitor this client for skin changes as secondary cancer may occur with chemotherapy.

Once again your most important role is to pay attention to any skin lesion that looks suspicious. Encourage your client to report any suspicious lesion to a physician. Early warning leads to early detection. Early detection gives your client the best chance of a successful outcome.

This is one more reason to promote regular visits to the salon and to offer back facials and full body treatments.

But be careful— because this is one case where a treatment like lymphatic drainage can cause harm to your client.

NO LYMPHATIC DRAINAGE TREATMENTS TO ANY MELANOMA CLIENT EVEN AFTER RECOVERY

RECOMMEND SUN SCREENS

CHAPTER 4

Breast Cancer

Breast Cancer

I am sure that everyone has heard about breast cancer, and most of us know at least one woman who has survived this disease. It is the most talked about cancer. The public awareness campaign includes TV ads, public announcements by movie stars, charity events to promote research, 5K runs sponsored by major cosmetic companies and entertainment personalities, a pink ribbon shaped pin, even stamps. Yet I find that fear and personal discomfort make it a taboo topic for conversation and investigation.

It is interesting to me that breast enlargement is easily discussed but breast preservation, better yet life preservation, is a whispered secret in the corners of rooms. It might be that the information we received as children has left us paralyzed — so afraid that we choose to ignore breast cancer, hoping it will go away. You might have grown up in a society like mine where cancer was referred to euphemistically as a "package" or another nickname, but never by the word itself. It was feared because once you "got it", people believed it meant a death sentence. All that was left was to remain silent, wait and pray. Often back then, the patient was not told the nature of her disease by the physician or family in order to minimize suffering. You might think I am talking about the 1920's. I am talking about 1984 when my father was diagnosed with cancer and was not told.

192,000 new cases of breast cancer are diagnosed every year. Every year there are 42,000 deaths.

Breast cancer accounts for one third of all cancers in women. It is the second leading cause of death from cancer and is the leading cause of death in women aged 40 to 55.

In order to understand breast cancer, it helps to know the breast structure, how the cancer develops and what factors influence the female breast.

The breast is made of a nipple, which is the external open end of tubes, also called ducts. On the other side of the ducts are 15 to 20 lobes, each one with a large number of lobules. At the end of each lobule are bulbs which can produce milk. The structure is like a tree with braches and leaves. All of this structure is surrounded by fat tissue, blood vessels and lymph nodes. There is no muscle tissue inside the breast. The muscles that support the breast are located beneath the breast above the ribs. The breast's function is to produce milk in order to feed the newborn baby.

The first stage of breast development occurs when a female embryo is 10-12 weeks old.

The second phase of development occurs at puberty. The hormone estrogen plays a major role in breast development, but in order to achieve complete breast development, an intricate balance of numerous hormones needs to be in place. With the increase of estrogen the following external changes are seen — a darkening of the nipples and an increase in the size of the breast. Internally there is a differentiation of the single cord or steam. Epithelial milk secreting cells are developing in the end of the capillary milk ducts, all connecting to the intra-lobular duct. It now looks like a tree with branches and few buds at the end of the branches.

At this stage the milk producing system is developed but is not yet capable of producing milk. These milk producing cells mature only in the third stage, pregnancy. The picture at this point is similar to a tree full of leaves.

Since estrogen is bonding to the breast tissue, breast size and tenderness fluctuate with the change of hormone levels during the normal menstrual cycle.

Breast cancer starts with a single epithelial cell lining the milk ducts; it is called Ductal Carcinoma, the most common breast cancer.

Breast cancer can also start in the lobules of the breast, which goes through a mutation, changing into a cancerous cell, Lobular Carcinoma. It grows and breaks through the membrane, then it spreads to the lymph nodes under the arm and from there to other organs like the lungs, liver and ultimately to the rest of the body. It can spread through the blood, and it can also invade the muscle tissue and the bones, moving into the chest cavity.

Risk Factors

Risk factors predict the likelihood of cancer to occur. This does not make it a 100% certainty that if you have the risk factor you will get cancer. It just says that you are more likely to get it than people without the risk factor. People with risk factors need to be monitored closely. It is important to know that over 70% of all breast cancers occur in women with no identifiable risk factor.

Where You Live

If you look at women in North America under the age of 80 you will find that one out of every nine women will get breast cancer. In Asia only 1 to 2 women out of 100 will get breast cancer. But when women from Japan move to Hawaii or the US mainland, they will be as likely to get breast cancer as any other American woman. This points out that genetics is not the sole cause of breast cancer and leads to the conclusion that the environment plays a role in increasing the likelihood of getting the disease. Increase in weight due to the American diet and the ease of life is one such factor, although at this point there is no evidence of a direct link between fat in the diet or any other food and breast cancer. What is known is that the more fat a women has in her body, particularly in the abdomen, the higher the levels of estrogen in the blood.

Urban living is listed as a risk for developing breast cancer. It is not clear if the reasons are stress and tension, easier physical life or pollution, but the fact is that a woman living in a city is more likely to get breast cancer than the one living on a farm or a small village.

Age

The older the woman, the more likely she will get breast cancer. The risk is greater after menopause.

The Estrogen Influence

A connection to the levels of estrogen and breast cancer is seen in three major events in a woman's maturing cycle and in other situations where estrogen is present. The first is menses. The older the woman when menses occurs, the less likely she is to get breast cancer. So a girl who menstruates by the age of 12 is more likely to get breast cancer than the girl who menstruates at age 14 or 16. It is somewhat ironic that girls who starve themselves at a young age, delaying the arrival of normal development and menses, also decrease their likelihood of getting breast cancer later in life.

The second major event is pregnancy. The woman who gives birth to a baby before she is 18, has less chance of getting breast cancer. A woman who becomes pregnant at the age of 30 or older increases her likelihood of getting breast cancer.

The third event is menopause. The average age of menopause in North America is 52. Late menopause after the age of 55 increases the risk. Early menopause due to natural causes or because of surgery decreases the risk.

HRT Hormonal Replacement Therapy

Research shows that women who take HRT for a long period of time have a small, but statistically significant risk of developing breast cancer. HRT also increases breast density, making it harder to detect breast cancer in early stages.

Birth Control Pills

There is a small risk increase for breast cancer that lasts up to ten years after a woman has stopped taking birth control pills. This is important, especially for women who have other risk factors.

DES (diethylstilbestrol)

Women who took DES have an increased risk of developing breast cancer. DES is a synthetic estrogen that was given to pregnant women between the years 1940 and 1971 to treat pregnancy complications and to prevent miscarriages. There is still not enough data to determine if the daughters born to these women also carry this risk.

Structure of the Breast or Breast Density

When the tissue in the breast is dense it is hard for a mammogram to detect breast cancer. Interestingly, the density in the tissue is from a large number of lobules and ducts, the type of tissue that breast cancer will develop in, and not from fat tissue in the breast. Women with dense breasts might want to ask for a breast ultrasound test. This test has a higher sensitivity.

Exercise

We all know that physical activity is important to our health. A clear connection is apparent with the risk of breast cancer. Lack of exercise will increase the risk of breast cancer.

Smoking

Cigarettes are carcinogens. Women smoking cigarettes are prone not only to lung cancer, but also to most types of cancer, including breast cancer. Women exposed to second hand cigarette smoke are also at increased risk.

Alcohol

One drink every day will increase the risk of breast cancer by 60%.

Radiation

Women exposed to radiation of the breast at a young age are at high risk for developing breast cancer.

Personal History

A woman with cancer in one breast is at high risk of getting the disease in the other breast.

Family History

A woman with a first degree female relative with breast cancer, like a mother, a sister or a daughter, especially if the relative had it at a young age, is at high risk of getting breast cancer.

Genetics

At least two genes are identified with a high potential to develop early breast cancer. They are BCRA 1 and BCRA 2. Although these defected genes are only found in about 25% of all women under 35 with breast cancer, those who do have these genes are at high risk. For example, if the damaged BRCA 1 gene is found, the risk is one out of two, in comparison to the general population's risk of one out of nine, and even less in a young age.

When BRCA 2 is found damaged, the risk is 37%. It is interesting, the damaged BCRA gene can be passed on to the daughter from either parent.

In general only 0.1%, or one out of one thousand people, has the damaged BCRA gene. The number increases to 2.3% or 23 out of a thousand, in Eastern European Jewish women.

The other genes that have been found to have a connection to breast cancer are BRCA3, p53, and NOEY2.

EARLY DETECTION IS THE KEY TO SURVIVAL

Survival

Survival of early stage localized breast cancer for five years has increased 18% in the past 60 years. In the 1940's the rate was 78%. It is currently 96%. If the cancer has spread survival goes down to 71%. If the cancer has metastased, only 18% will survive for 5 years.

The key is early detection. Despite all the controversy, the facts show that every woman, including the one with no family history or known risk factors, should have a mammogram every year from the age of 40 for the rest of her life. A mammogram will detect breast cancer on an average 1.7 years before it can be felt with a manual breast exam.

Medical Treatment

The treatment of breast cancer depends of the type of cancer, its stage, the age of the woman, her health and if the cancer has receptors that are sensitive to hormones or not. The goal is to eradicate all cancerous cells.

Surgery

Surgery is almost always indicated. The extent of the surgery depends on how much the cancer has spread. In addition to removal of the breast tissue, some or all of the lymph nodes are removed. When needed, the entire breast and muscles are removed.

Radiation

External radiation is given to the breast at the tumor site. Radiation therapy is based on the knowledge that living cells exposed to high energy will be damaged and not be able to multiply. The second fact that makes radiation therapy work is that cancerous cells multiply at a higher rate then normal cells. The result is that radiation is able to damage the rapidly multiplying cancerous cells while limiting the damage to healthy cells.

There are different types of radiation therapy. The most common one is from an outside source. The energy used is X-ray, cobalt-60 gamma ray, electron beam, neutron beam or proton beam. The beam is directed at the tumor site on the body. The treatment is given every day for several weeks. The time of the exposure is short to minimize damage to the surrounding healthy tissue. If the patient's overall health allows it, she can go home and continue with regular activities when the treatment is concluded.

Side Effects of Radiation

Lack of energy is the most noticeable side effect of radiation therapy because the body is trying to heal the damaged cells. Nausea, vomiting, change of taste in the mouth and loss of appetite can also occur. Most side effects will disappear with the end of treatment.

Skin Reactions to Radiation

Skin reaction is usually delayed and can be seen two weeks or more after radiation has begun because the damage that is done by radiation to the cell is only pronounced when the cell divides. The reaction can vary from red skin, swelling, itching or dry skin that is scaling. Sometimes the skin will look like it has been burned and might ulcerate. In most cases the skin will get hyper pigmented.

Some people will develop wet skin, particularly in areas were there are skin folds. Since the skin is moist, it breaks easily which increases the danger of infection.

The patient should wear pure cotton and avoid tight clothing. Itching or scratching of the irritated skin should be avoided at all costs.

No heating or cooling of the site is allowed without consulting the treating physician. Do not apply any covering or bandages to the radiated site.

Chemotherapy

Advanced chemotherapy is used to treat breast cancer.

Chemotherapy is the popular name for the treatment of cancer with drugs. This group of drugs is also called Antineoplastic agents: anti meaning against, neoplastic meaning cancer. They are also called Cytotoxic: cyto meaning cell, toxic meaning poison.

The job of chemotherapy drugs is to kill cells. They are effective against cells that divide rapidly. Normal cells limit their division; cancer cells, having lost that ability, keep on multiplying and growing.

The skin and the digestive system are designed to self heal which is why their normal cells multiply at a higher rate. Even though they may be healthy, they will be affected by chemotherapy. When I talk about the skin with regard to chemotherapy, I include hair and nails. When I refer to the digestive system I include the inside of the mouth and the stomach.

Chemotherapy is administered in order to eliminate the tumor, to reduce the tumor size so it can be removed by surgery or to shrink the cancer in order to reduce the tumor's effects. For example, the effect of a tumor pressing on a nerve is often pain

Chemotherapy treatment is given orally as a tablet, intravenously as an injection into the vein by a catheter into the site of the cancer.

The treatment is given in a series of courses where the medication is taken for a period of time, then stopped to allow the healthy cells to recuperate. Treatment can be six months or longer, depending on the cancer.

Side Effects Of Chemotherapy

Note: The side effects listed here are the ones I think you need to be aware of for your practice. There are many additional side effects that are life threatening, like damage to the liver, kidneys, and lungs. Side effects have been recorded as many as 17 years after the completion of chemotherapy. The secondary cancer risk is another major problem, as any medication that cures cancer has the potential to cause cancer.

Chemotherapy is the most aggressive drug treatment known and has severe side effects. There is a delayed appearance of the side effects. Side effects will appear when the cells start dying. Tiredness or total exhaustion are common side effects because the body needs all its energy to eliminate the damaging chemicals and to heal. Nausea and vomiting will occur and can be treated with medications.

Chemotherapy affects the blood system. Clotting, known as thrombocytopenia, is a common side effect. On the other end of the spectrum excessive bleeding can also result.

Another result of chemotherapy is that veins can appear darker. It is most noticeable with darker skinned people. This will reverse itself once the drugs are eliminated from the body.

Reduction in the function of the immune system makes it easy for chemotherapy patients to become infected.

Nerve and muscle damage can appear as weakness, loss of balance, pain, tingling, burning or even numbness and loss of sensation in the hands and feet. These effects can last up to one year after chemotherapy has ended.

Depression is common. It is a reaction to the chemotherapy, the cancer itself and fear of death.

Skin Reactions

Alopecia, the loss of hair from the scalp and from the entire body including the eyebrows and eyelashes, is one of the effects women fear most. Hair will come back once chemotherapy is over; however, it might come back in a different color and or texture.

The nails can become thin and brittle with vertical lines and cracks. They may also become dark or yellow.

Skin will become sensitive, thin and will get infected easily. Skin can become dry and itchy and will be sensitive to sun. Some chemotherapy medications are phototoxic. Pre-existing conditions like acne or psoriasis may reappear.

When a patient is receiving chemotherapy the skin site of previous radiation or burn can become red, and the skin can blister and peel. This can last anywhere from a few hours to several days. This reaction is called " Radiation recall".

If the chemotherapy leaks or touches the skin where the IV is inserted, pain and ulceration will occur. It might require a plastic surgery correction.

Bone Marrow Transplant

When breast cancer has spread to other organs, higher doses of chemotherapy might be needed. These potent chemotherapy doses will compromise the woman's own bone marrow. If this is the case then a bone marrow transplant will be performed to help with recovery.

Bone marrow transplant is a generic term that includes the harvesting of different stem cells and transplanting them. The stem cells that produce blood and immune cells are located in the bone marrow. This procedure increases the quantity of the desired stem cells, and as a result, a larger number of healthy cells will be produced.

A bone marrow transplant is done when the stem cells are malignant or when there are not enough stem cells because they have been killed with high doses of radiation or chemotherapy. Bone marrow can be frozen and thawed making this procedure readily available. Once marrow is located, it is aspirated from the posterior or anterior iliac crest. It is cleaned and processed then infused into the chest bone.

There are two sources of bone marrow. Bone marrow can be obtained from the patient's own marrow, which is called autologous. Bone marrow can be taken from another person, a donor; this is referred to as allogenic. The donor can be a family member or not.

The probability that a non-family member will be a match is only about 1 in 10,000. In the US there is a National Marrow Donor Program with more then 3 million volunteers. It takes three to four months to find a match. Today, about half of all transplant patients find a match through this program. The chances of finding a match with a family member are better than 50%.

Side Effects

The problem with a bone marrow transplant is rejection. When the marrow transplant uses the patient's own bone marrow there is no problem. If the patient is lucky enough to have an identical twin there will also be no problem with rejection. But with a family member or an unrelated donor, there can be a rejection. To overcome the possibility of rejection, the patient is given medications, like corticosteroids, that shut down the immune system. This makes the patient susceptible to infections.

The first 3 months after the transplant are critical, but some patients require medication for up to three years after the transplant. Because of the risk of infections, antibiotics and anti-viral medications are also prescribed. The first sign of a problem will be the appearance of a rash.

Prednisone

Prednisone will be given in the case of a donor bone marrow transplant. Prednisone, a corticosteroid, is a potent drug. It is prescribed for cancer patients to reduce swelling, tumor size and to prevent rejection of the bone marrow transplant.

Depending on the condition, a patient can take it for a week or for years, as is the case with bone marrow transplants.

As with any potent drug, Prednisone has many side effects. Three affect the skin directly; skin thinning, healing time reduction and infection masking.

Skin Thinning

Dermal atrophy (thinning of the skin) makes the need for exfoliating services or ingredients absolutely unnecessary. The skin is already thin because of the medication, and it heals slowly. You need to avoid: AHA, BHA, Vitamin A and Vitamin C in high concentrations. It also makes waxing hair removal unsafe for a period of 6 months from the time Prednisone treatment ended.

Infection Masking

Masking of infections occurs because Prednisone reduces the inflammation, redness and itchiness associated with the infection process. Although you may not see clear symptoms, the infection is still evolving.

Because of the increased sensitivity to infections and the effect of masking, it is a good idea to use extra precaution. Make sure your equipment and products are clean so you will not cause infection.

If your client suffers from acne, psoriasis or rosacea you may see a flare up while she is being treated with Prednisone or when she gets off the medication.

You can also see steroidal acne from Prednisone (it can be diagnosed by the dermatologist). Conventional salon treatments or cosmetic ingredients can reduce the redness or irritation, but this problem will not go away until the Medication is stopped.

Other Side Effects

It is unfortunate that women who take Prednisone for a long period of time will develop dark course facial hair, similar to a man's. On the other hand, they may experience Alopecia (loss of hair on the head).

Because of potential increased blood pressure and fluid retention you should avoid salon treatments that stimulate blood flow to the heart.

Immune busters

A new approach to treat breast cancer is the use of immune busters in concert with chemotherapy to enhance the body's own cancer fighting abilities. (see page 28)

Hormonal Therapy

When a breast cancer has receptors that are sensitive to estrogen it is called an Estrogen Receptor - positive tumor - ER-positive. When the tumor has no sensitivity to estrogen it is called ER-negative.

ER-positive cancers are easier to treat. If the cancer is sensitive to hormones, the ovaries might be removed to eliminate the production of estrogen. If the woman has had her ovaries removed pre-menopause, she will go into immediate menopause. Medications like Tamoxifen, that block the estrogen receptors, will be used both to stop the tumor from growing and to prevent recurrence of the cancer.

Tamoxifen

Tamoxifen, sold under the brand name Nolvadex, is a drug being prescribed to prevent breast cancer. Tamoxifen is an antiestrogen drug that is prescribed for women following surgery for breast cancer. It is used in conjunction with chemotherapy or radiation. A five year study indicates that women who took Tamoxifen were forty-five percent less likely to develop cancer than women who did not. However, the study also indicated that there are two known side effects of Tamoxifen— uterine cancer and blood clots.

When a client suffers from blood clots, you should avoid body wraps or massage to the lower extremities because these treatments increase the risk of blood clots traveling to the heart and lungs which could create a life-threatening situation.

Note: Massage therapy can be beneficial in preventing blood clots. In some women nausea and vomiting can be induced by fragrances, pressure to the chest, and/or pressure to the abdominal area. Women taking Tamoxifen also experience a higher rate of hot flashes. Edema, skin rashes and dry skin can also result. If the client suffers from dry skin be sure and use appropriate creams.

Dizziness, headaches, depression, confusion, fatigue and muscle cramps have also been reported by users of Tamoxifin

Salon Treatments

DON'T ever use products containing hormones on women who have had breast cancer.

Salon Treatment of Radiation Therapy Clients

CELLS WITHOUT OXYGEN ARE NOT AFFECTED BY RADIATION. WHILE YOUR CLIENT IS GOING THROUGH RADIATION TREATMENT, DO NOT USE ANY OXYGEN TREATMENTS, OXYGEN CREAMS, OR OXYGEN BARS. THEY WILL INTERFERE WITH THE RADIATION TREATMENT.

IT IS IMPORTANT THAT YOU DO NOT REMOVE OR TOUCH ANY MARKINGS ON THE SKIN AS THEY ARE RADIATION GUIDES

While undergoing radiation therapy the patient is highly advised to consult only the treating physician or nurse about skin care, including the type of soap, lotion, powder, deodorant or even sunscreen to use. The skin needs to be protected from the sun, but sunscreens can interfere with the effectiveness of the radiation. The physician needs to be consulted about the use of sunscreens.

No hair removal is allowed at the site and no depilatory lotions. If hair needs to be removed, use an electric shaver, but consult the doctor first. As for hair removal on other parts of the body, consult the physician first.

It is important to know that only mild liquid cleanser and moisturizer with no heavy metals should be used by the client. Remember the skin is susceptible to infections. Creams or lotions should be water based and should not contain Vaseline (petrolatum or mineral oil) because petrolatum or mineral oil can create a barrier that prevents the skin from breathing, trapping moisture and bacteria, thus increasing the risk of infection. Silicones like Dimethicone are good ingredients at this stage. Vitamins, antioxidants, oxygen, peroxide, perfume and any irritating ingredient should be avoided because they can interfere with the radiation treatment. No lotion should be applied within two hours of radiation therapy.

Salon Treatment The First Two Years After Radiation Therapy

After radiation therapy ends the use of vitamin E and silicones can be beneficial to the recovery of the skin at the site of the radiation. At this point you're treating skin that has been severely burned. Consult the physician before any treatment. Do not attempt to lighten the skin or to fight the hyperpigmentation. In time it should fade away.

Do not try to erase the radiation site markings because they might be tattoos. Avoid any aggressive treatment and any exfoliating or anti-aging treatment anywhere on the body.

Recommend supportive skin care and sun screen. Clients who have undergone radiation treatments are more susceptible to skin cancer. The radiation site can be sensitive for a long time. Be careful when treating the skin in that area. In some patients a chronic skin reaction may occur at the radiation treatment site after six to twelve months. The skin will be thin and easy to break or irritate. Scar tissue may develop under the epidermis. Permanent loss of hair at the site of treatment may occur.

Salon Treatment Two Years Or More After Radiation Therapy

If no other health conditions exist you can resume regular treatments two years after the end of radiation treatment. Radiation patients are more prone to develop skin cancers, so you need to monitor this client for any skin lesions or skin changes.

Finally, as the population ages, you will be treating more and more people who have undergone radiation therapy. Now is a good time to get involved with the cancer center in your area. You might be able to work with the nurse or doctor in providing skin care to their patients.

Salon Treatments For Chemotherapy Clients
While on chemotherapy and up to 2 years post treatment.

Before treating this client check with her treating doctor.

Patients are urged by their medical care givers to continue their normal life as part of the overall goal of maintaining a positive attitude to fight and overcome the cancer.

If you choose, you can get involved with your local cancer treatment center and become an integral part of the cancer support system.

Your salon or spa can become a place of refuge and provide a bit of normal routine in a crisis situation. Here are some do's and don'ts.

DO use extra precaution because these clients tend to get infected easily. Avoid any service with the potential to compromise the skin's integrity: such as extraction, deep cleaning, hair removal by waxing, sugaring, threading or tweezing.

DO use only clean products and pay special attention to prevent cross contamination.

DO use a mouth mask, especially if you have been near anyone who is sick or with a cold.

DO use products that are gentle, preferably without perfumes and alcohol.

DO use moisturizing creams and lotions beacuse the skin is dry and thin. Some beneficial ingredients are starches from oatmeal, rice, or corn, silicones like Dimethicone, Aloe Vera, chamomile and zinc oxide.

DO recommend a good sun screen of at least SPF 15.

DO recommend a nail strengthener and administer a hand moisturizing treatment with warm oil. Olive oil and almond oil are beneficial.

DO help your client to get off the treatment table to prevent any falls.

DON'T peel or exfoliate the skin. Do not use chemical or botanical/organic ingredients that thin the skin including AHA, BHA, vitamin A or C. Do not use microdermabrasion or scrubs.

DON'T use any ingredients that have the potential to be absorbed into the skin.

DON'T use any heating masks or extreme cold treatments

DON'T use body treatments like body wraps and massage of the legs because of the risk of blood clot.

DON'T suggest or recommend any oral vitamins , food supplements or any herbal remedies

DON'T use essential oils.

Make Up

Because of hair loss, including eyebrows and lashes, your client might need your help. You can teach her how to enhance her appearance, but do not use any permanent make up. Because of the danger of infection, remind her to start with new make up and brushes. Recommend products that are water soluble, that are easily removed with water, containing titanium dioxide.

Salon Treatment Two Years After Chemotherapy Is Completed.

If there are no other conditions you can treat the skin as needed. Remember even after two years, the skin can be extremely sensitive and thin. Monitor this client for skin changes as secondary cancer may occur with chemotherapy.

Bone marrow

Before treating a client who has had a bone marrow transplant consult the treating doctor. If the client has taken corticosteroids like Prednisone in the two year period after the treatment ends, the skin will be thin, slow to heal and susceptible to infection.

Prednisone

If your client is taking prednisone or she is in the first six months after treatment has ceased:

DON'T use any skin thinning treatments including microdermabrasion, and anti-aging treatments, AHAs, BHAs, Vitamin A, Vitamin C serums.

DON'T remove hair by waxing until 6 months after Prednisone medication has ceased.

DON'T use treatments that increase blood flow to the heart.

DO use skin care treatment that is gentle and supportive to the skin.
DO encourage your client to wear sunscreen.

After two years

You can resume regular skin treatments two years after the end of all medical treatments related to the bone marrow transplant if no other medical conditions exist.

Lymphectomy

Most patients will have had some lymph nodes or all lymph nodes removed from under the arm on the same side as the breast cancer. This not only causes pain and sensitivity in the arm and shoulder, it causes a problem with proper lymphatic drainage. A condition called lymph edema where the arm gets swollen can evolve and become a danger to the patient's well being. This condition can be prevented with the proper treatment. This is one more place where you can help.

It is important to know that because of the elimination of the lymph nodes, no proper drainage is available in the arm, making it sensitive to infections for the rest of the client's life. This is why it is important for you to be very careful with your client's arm making sure it does not get infected. The client should also avoid putting pressure on this arm. For example, pressure created by carrying her purse should be avoided. The use of gloves when washing dishes and working in the garden is a common recommendation for infection prevention.

Exercise of the arm is important as is careful treatment to prevent any assault to the hand and arm.

Manual lymphatic drainage can be of help. There are also machines which perform lymphatic drainage. But before treating you should consult the physician to see if the treatment is appropriate. If it is, ask the physician about recommended duration, method and frequency.

Avoid any procedure that might compromise the integrity of the skin of this hand, arm and shoulder for the rest of your client's life. This include manicures. Do not use any sharp tools that can injure the skin. Hair removal by waxing or sugaring on or under the arm should not be performed.

Consult the physician before attempting any body wraps, Vichy Showers, massage or cellulite treatment and avoid any extreme heat or cold on this arm and shoulder. This includes wet and dry sauna.

Products containing ingredients that are absorbed into the body like vitamin A and essential oils should be avoided on the hand, arm and shoulder where the lymphectomy was performed.

Make your client comfortable when on a facial bed by elevating the arm. Rest it and the shoulder on a supportive pillow.

CALL THE TREATING PHYSICIAN BEFORE YOU ADMINISTER ANY SALON TREATMENT TO A CANCER PATIENT, A RECOVERING CANCER PATIENT OR A FORMER CANCER PATIENT.

CHAPTER 5

Cervical Cancer

Cervical Cancer

Cervical cancer is one more example of how important it is to do all the yearly tests because if cervical cancer is detected early, it can be cured.

In a time when alternative medicine is growing stronger and louder voices are heard speaking against conventional medicine this is yet another example of the importance of seeing the doctor for a checkup at least once a year.

Description and epidimiology

The Cervix is a column shaped structure that connects the vagina to the womb (uterus).

The cells lining that hollow column can become abnormal and then cancerous. There are several types of cancer of the cervix but the majority of cancer cases occur in the thin flat cells that line the surface of the cervix. Those cells are Squamous cells and the cancer is called Squamous Cell Carcinoma.

When abnormal cells are found they are classified as Squamous Intraepithelial Lesion (SIL), Low Grade or High Grade. The Low Grade is the early stage change in the cell with a small number of abnormal cells. Sometimes a reversal can happen naturally, and these cells disappear. But in other cases the lesion can grow larger and become High Grade. Other names for Low grade SIL are mild dysplasia or cervical intraepithelial neoplasia 1 (CIN1).

In High grade SIL, also known as severe dysplasia CIN2, CIN3 or carcinoma in situ, the cells are distinctly different from the normal cells and the quantity of abnormal cells is greater than in Low grade. The good news is that at this stage the lesion is still localized, and it will take months to years before the cells become cancerous and start spreading. The cancerous cells spread deeper into the cervix consequently spreading to nearby organs like the uterus, ovaries, rectum, bladder, bones and spine even into the lungs via the lymphatic system and the blood vessels.

There are usually no symptoms until the cells become cancerous. Symptoms include irregular bleeding and bleeding after intercourse. Pain in the lower back appears in the advanced stage of cervical cancer.

Thirty years ago cervical cancer was the cancer that killed most women. But today it is the cancer that is the easiest to detect early by a relatively easy test, the Pap smear, and by a pelvic exam. Once detected, it can be treated and eliminated before spreading.

Despite this fact, in the US there are about 15,000 new cases of cervical cancer every year. In the year 2000, 4,600 women died from the spread of this cancer. It is worth noting that 85% of the deceased women never had a Pap smear. Remember, Pap smears detect more then 50,000 cases of early stage cervical cancer every year.

The Pap Smear

The full name for Pap smear is Papanicolaou smear. The test is named after George Nicolaou (1883-1962), a Greek physician, anatomist and cytologist who developed the test.

Pap smears and pelvic exams are preformed by a gynecologist in an office or clinic. The doctor inserts a cotton swab moistened with saline, a wooden spatula, or a little brush into the cervix and scrapes a sample of the cells that line the cervix. He smears the sample onto a microscope glass. The sample is then sent to a laboratory where a cytologist analyzes it.

If abnormal cells are found further testing and examination by the doctor takes place. In order to minimize human error and increase test reliability the Pap smear test is constantly being improved by scientists.

Every woman over the age of 18, earlier if the women has had sexual relations, should get a Pap smear every year.

The Pelvic Exam

The pelvic exam is when the doctor feels the inside of the female organs and uses a speculum to look and see if there are any changes in the upper part of the vagina and cervix. The doctor can feel any changes to the female organs, the bladder and rectum, including any swelling, inflammation, change in texture, shape or size.

Risk Factors

Although many women have the risk factors it does not mean that they will get the disease. Scientists believe that the more risk factors a woman has - the higher the risk. Most experts believe that at least two risk factors need to be present in order for there to be any risk.

Sexual activity/number of partners

If a woman becomes sexually active before the age of 18 she is at higher risk for cervical cancer. The more sexually active a woman is with multipale partners, the higher her risk.

The more partners the man has the higher the risk for the woman. The theory is that Sexually Transmitted Diseases (STD) will cause changes in the cell structure, and women with high risk sexual practices run a higher risk of contracting STDs.

Birth Control Pills

This is a case of the chicken or the egg. It is not clear if because a woman takes BCP and is more sexually active THAT is why she is at risk, or is it the BCP hormones that put her at risk? There is no evidence that the hormones are the cause, but it is known that women who take BCP are at a higher risk.

Viruses

Human Papilloma (HPV) and genital herpes viruses do not cause cervical cancer by themselves but it is believed that when they occur together they trigger cellular abnormalities that can lead to cancer.

Smoking
The more cigarettes a woman smokes, the higher the risk. The more years she smokes the higher the risk.

DES
DES (Diethylstilbestrol) is a hormone that was given to women between 1940 and 1970 to prevent miscarriages. Daughters of mothers who took this hormone have a risk of developing a rare type of cervical cancer before the age of 19.

Compromised Immune System
If the immune system is weak because of medications or disease the risk of cervical cancer increases. For example people who have an organ transplant, chemotherapy or have HIV are more likely to develop this cancer.

Age
Most cases of cervical cancer occur in women over the age of 40.

Medical Treatments
Good news: if the problem is detected in the early stage where the cells are just abnormal, the disease can be cured. The treatment is localized and the abnormal cells are eliminated by freezing, cryosurgery, or burning, cauterization/ diathermy. Another way of burning the cells is with a laser. Surgery of conization = LEEP is when the lesion is removed by the doctor punching a cone like section into the cervix.

If the cells have progressed beyond the early stage, are high grade and the woman is at risk, a hysterectomy, a surgery to remove the uterus, can be performed.

The treatment of cervical cancer depends on the stage of the cancer. Protocol is surgery to remove the uterus plus radiation treatments.

Surgery

Surgery can be performed on the lining of the cervix, or it can include the uterus. In some cases a total hysterectomy will be performed where the cervix, uterus, fallopian tubes and ovaries will be removed. Lymph nodes will also be removed in the area close to the tumor. In this case the woman will go into early menopause.

If the patient is a young, pre-menopausal woman who has had her ovaries surgically removed she will experience the immediate onset of menopause. This is because her ovaries, the organs that produce estrogen and progesterone have been removed. The patient may suffer hot flashes and the skin will go into an early aging process.

Radiation

Radiation can be external, internal or implant radiation, where a radioactive capsule is inserted into the cervix for one to three days. This is repeated for one to two weeks.

What is Radiation therapy? Radiation therapy is based on the knowledge that living cells exposed to high energy will be damaged and not be able to multiply. The second fact that makes radiation therapy work is that cancerous cells multiply at a higher rate then normal cells. The result is that radiation is able to damage the rapidly multiplying cancerous cells while limiting the damage to healthy cells.

There are different types of radiation therapy. The most common one is from an outside source. The energy used is X-ray, cobalt-60 gamma ray, electron beam, neutron beam or proton beam. The beam is directed at the tumor site on the body. The treatment is given every day for several weeks. The time of the exposure is short to minimize damage to the surrounding healthy tissue. If the patient's overall health allows it, she can go home and continue with regular activities when the treatment is concluded.

Remote Brachytherapy is another type of radiation treatment which is done with an outside source of radiation that is directed through a catheter or tube directly to the tumor. This is considered an inside therapy as the beam is delivered directly into the tumor.

Another type of internal radiation is when the source of energy is implanted inside the tumor or in the area where the tumor has been removed.

A variation of this treatment is when the source is not encapsulated, but the radioactive material is injected into the body. Since the radioactive material is in the body, the patient is radioactive and needs to be isolated in the hospital. Visitors and medical personal are limited to short visits so they will not be affected by the radiation.

Side Effects of Radiation

Lack of energy is the most noticeable side effect of radiation therapy because the body is trying to heal the damaged cells. Nausea, vomiting, change of taste in the mouth and loss of appetite can also occur. Most side effects will disappear with the end of treatment.

Skin Reactions to Radiation

Skin reaction is usually delayed and can be seen after two weeks or more after radiation has begun because the damage that is done by radiation to the cell is only pronounced when the cell divides. The reaction can vary from red skin, swelling, itching, to dry skin that is scaling. Sometimes the skin will look like it has been burned and might ulcerate. In most cases the skin will get hyper pigmented.

Some people will develop wet skin, particularly in areas were there are skin folds. Since the skin is moist, it breaks easily which increases the danger of infection.

The patient should wear pure cotton and avoid tight clothing. Itching or scratching of the irritated skin should be avoided at all costs. No heating or cooling of the site is allowed without consulting the treating physician. Do not apply any covering or bandages to the radiated site.

Salon Treatments

Salon Treatments of Radiation Therapy Clients

CELLS WITHOUT OXYGEN ARE NOT AFFECTED BY RADIATION. WHILE YOUR CLIENT IS GOING THROUGH RADIATION TREATMENT, DO NOT USE ANY OXYGEN TREATMENTS, OXYGEN CREAMS, OR OXYGEN BARS. THEY WILL INTERFERE WITH THE RADIATION TREATMENT.

IT IS IMPORTANT THAT YOU DO NOT REMOVE OR TOUCH ANY MARKINGS ON THE SKIN AS THEY ARE RADIATION GUIDES.

While undergoing radiation therapy the patient is highly advised to consult only the treating physician or nurse about skin care, including the type of soap, lotion, powder, deodorant or even sunscreen to use. The skin needs to be protected from the sun, but sunscreens can interfere with the effectiveness of the radiation. The physician needs to be consulted about the use of sunscreens.

No hair removal is allowed at the site and no depilatory lotions. If hair needs to be removed, use an electric shaver, but consult the doctor first. As for hair removal on other parts of the body consult the physician first.

It is important to know that only mild liquid cleanser and moisturizer without heavy metals should be used by the client. Remember the skin is susceptible to infections. Creams or lotions should be water based and should not contain Vaseline (petrolatum or mineral oil) because they can create a barrier that prevents the skin from breathing, trapping moisture and bacteria thus increasing the risk of infection. Silicones like Dimethicone are good ingredients at this stage. Vitamins, antioxidants, oxygen, peroxide, perfume and any irritating ingredient should be avoided because they can interfere with the radiation treatment. No lotion should be applied within two hours of radiation therapy.

Salon Treatment The First Two Years After Radiation Therapy

After radiation therapy ends the use of vitamin E and silicones can be beneficial to the recovery of the skin at the site of the radiation. At this point you're treating skin that has been severely burned. Consult the physician before any treatment. Do not attempt to lighten the skin or to fight the hyper pigmentation. In time it should fade away.

Do not try to erase the radiation site markings because they might be tattoos. Avoid any aggressive treatment and any exfoliating or anti-aging treatment anywhere on the body. Recommend supportive skin care and sun screen. Clients who have undergone radiation treatments are more susceptible to skin cancer. The site of the radiation can be sensitive for a long time. Be careful when treating the skin in that area. In some patients a chronic skin reaction may occur at the site of radiation after six to twelve months. The skin will be thin and easy to break or irritate. Scar tissue may develop under the epidermis. Permanent loss of hair at the site of treatment may occur.

Salon Treatment Two Years Or More After Radiation Therapy

If no other health conditions exist you can resume regular treatments two years after the end of radiation treatment. Radiation patients are more prone to develop skin cancers, so you need to monitor this client for any skin lesions or skin changes. Please see the Skin Cancer Chapter.

Finally, as the population ages, you will be treating more and more people who have undergone radiation therapy. Now is a good time to get involved with the cancer center in your area. You might be able to work with the nurse or doctor in providing skin care to their patients.

CALL THE TREATING PHYSICIAN BEFORE YOU ADMINISTER ANY SALON TREATMENT TO A CANCER PATIENT, A RECOVERING CANCER PATIENT OR A FORMER CANCER PATIENT.

CHAPTER 6

Uterine Cancer

Uterine Cancer

The uterus is a female reproductive organ. Its job is to receive the fertilized egg and to provide the necessary environment for the embryo's development.

The uterus is located above the cervix and between the bladder in the front and the rectum in the back. It is shaped like a pear standing on its head with the narrow side connected to the cervix.

The upper side, fundus, is connected to the fallopian tubes on each side. It is a hollow structure with the bulk of it, called the body or corpus, on top. The uterus, when not in pregnancy condition, is 6.5 cm long, 3.5cm wide, and 2.5cm thick. It has two important layers. The outer layer is a smooth muscle layer called the myometrium and the inner layer is called the endometrium.

The endometrium is the layer that prepares itself for the fertile egg. It starts changing every month when estrogen is secreted from the ovaries. The endometrium swells and builds up and becomes as thick as 5 cm. When no fertilization occurs the endomitrium breaks down and menstrual bleeding appears. The endometrium goes through this monthly cycle of building and breaking down from puberty until menopause. At menopause the endomitrium atrophies.

The endometrium is the layer of the uterus where most cancers develop. It is the layer that has a rapid cell turnover. Carcinoma of the endometrium is the most common cancer of the reproduction organs. More than 36,000 cases are diagnosed yearly. Because of the structure of the uterus, cancer in the uterus will exhibit symptoms even at an early stage. This is why most cases are found in the early stages when the cancer is localized, making uterine cancer number 7 on the list of death causing cancers. 6,500 deaths a year are attributed to uterine cancer.

The common symptoms of uterine cancer are unusual bleeding

or discharge, pain during urination or intercourse and pain in the area of the pelvis. These can also be the symptoms of other non-cancerous conditions, but any woman who experiences any of these symptoms should get checked by a doctor.

Most uterine cancers occur in post menopausal women, but 25% of all cases are found in women younger than 50, and 5% in women younger than 40. Uterine cancer is common in the US and Eastern Europe and is rare in Asia.

The endometrium can develop fibroids inside or benign tissue growth outside of the uterus, called Endometriosis. They are not cancers and do not evolve into cancer. A condition where there is an increased number of cells in the lining of the uterus is called en-dometrial hyperplasia. It can develop into cancer.

Uterine cancer, when not detected early, can spread through the lymph nodes and the blood vessels to other organs of the body like the lungs, liver and bone. Another type of uterine cancer can develop in the muscle layer of the uterus, myometrium, and is called uterine sarcoma. It is rare, and this chapter does not cover this cancer.

Risk Factors
Age
Women over 50 are at greater risk. Although most cases occur after menopause, prior to menopause there is also risk.

Endometrial Hyperplasia (see above)

Estrogen Exposure
The longer the uterus is exposed to estrogen the more likely a woman is to get uterine cancer. The younger the woman when she begins menstruating, the higher the risk. The older a woman is when she hits menopause, the higher the risk. If the woman has had no children her risk is higher.

This also explains the next three risk factors:

Hormonal Replacement Therapy (HRT)

Women who take HRT after menopause are at a higher risk for uterine cancer. The risk is higher when women take estrogen replacement without progesterone. There is a correlation between the dosage and the length of treatment: the higher the dose and the longer the treatment - the higher the risk. In menopausal women the uterus is exposed to prescription estrogen when nature intended the uterus to be atrophied and resting.

Tamoxifen

Tamoxifen is a drug taken to prevent or oppose breast cancer. It has estrogen like properties, putting the uterus at risk of developing cancer. This is one of those "walking a thin line" medications where the benefits outweigh the risks.

Obesity

Fatty tissue, particularly in the abdomen and thighs, produces estrogen. Women with more fat in their body will have higher estrogen levels. This explains why women who are over weight have a higher risk of developing cancer of the uterus.

Race

White women are at a higher risk than African American women.

Medical Treatment of Uterine Cancer

Diagnosis and prevention are done by pelvic exam, pap test, transvaginal ultrasound and a biopsy to clarify the diagnosis.

Treatment depends on how far the cancer has spread. This is an evaluation done by the doctor and is called staging. Four stages are recognized in the spread of uterine cancer:

Stage 1 The cancer is in the uterus.

Stage 2 The cancer spreads to the cervix

Stage 3 The cancer spreads outside the uterus, but not outside the pelvis, and there is no spreading to the bladder or rectum. Lymph nodes can be affected.

Stage 4 The cancer spreads to the bladder, rectum or beyond the pelvis.

Surgery is almost always performed. It entails removal of the uterus, cervix, vaginal tissue, ovaries and some lymph nodes depending on where the cancer has spread.

If the patient is a young premenopausal woman, and her ovaries have been removed by surgery, she will experience the immediate onset of menopause. This is because the ovaries, the organs that produce estrogen and progesterone are removed. The patient may suffer hot flashes, and the skin will go into early aging process and may be dry.

Radiation Therapy

Radiation therapy can be given before or after surgery and will be external or internal. Radiation therapy is based on the knowledge that living cells exposed to high energy will be damaged and not be able to multiply. The second fact that makes radiation therapy work is that cancerous cells multiply at a higher rate than normal cells. The result is that radiation is able to damage the rapidly multiplying cancerous cells while limiting the damage to healthy cells.

There are different types of radiation therapy. The most common one is from an outside source. The energy used is X-ray, cobalt-60 gamma ray, electron beam, neutron beam or proton beam. The beam is directed at the tumor site on the body. The treatment is given every day for several weeks. The time of the exposure is short to minimize damage to the surrounding healthy tissue. If the patient's overall health allows it, she can go home and continue with regular activities when the treatment is concluded.

Remote Brachytherapy is another type of radiation treatment which is done with an outside source of radiation that is directed through a catheter or tube directly to the tumor. This is considered an inside therapy as the beam is delivered directly into the tumor.

Another type of internal radiation is when the source of energy is implanted inside the tumor or in the area where the tumor has been removed.

A variation of this treatment is when the source is not encapsulated but the radioactive material is injected into the body. Since the radioactive material is in the body, the patient is radioactive and needs to be isolated in the hospital. Visitors and medical personal are limited to short visits so they will not be affected by the radiation.

Side Effects of Radiation

Lack of energy is the most noticeable side effect of radiation therapy because the body is trying to heal the damaged cells. Nausea, vomiting, change of taste in the mouth and loss of appetite can also occur. Most side effects will disappear with the end of treatment.

Skin Reactions to Radiation

Skin reaction is usually delayed and can be seen after two weeks or longer from the start of radiation because the damage that is done by radiation to the cell is only pronounced when the cell divides. The reaction can vary from red skin, swelling, itching or dry skin that is scaling. Sometimes the skin will look like it has been burned and might ulcerate. In most cases the skin will get hyper pigmented.

Some people will develop wet skin, particularly in areas were there are skin folds. Since the skin is moist, it breaks easily increasing the danger of infection.

The patient should wear pure cotton and avoid tight clothing. Itching or scratching of the irritated skin should be avoided at all costs. No heating or cooling of the site is allowed without consulting the treating physician. Do not apply any covering or bandages to the radiated site.

Hormonal Therapy

When a woman cannot go through surgery or radiation, or when the cancer has spread to the lungs, hormonal therapy can be administered. Progesterone type medications are given orally when estrogen and progesterone receptors are found. The hormones are given to block the estrogen receptors of the cancer cells so they will not grow. The major side effects of progesterone are water retention, increased appetite and weight gain. Premenopausal women will also experience a change in their menstrual cycle.

Chemotherapy

Chemotherapy might be needed. Chemotherapy is the popular name for the treatment of cancer with drugs. This group of drugs is also called Antineoplastic agents: anti meaning against, neoplastic meaning cancer. They are also called Cytotoxic: cyto meaning cell and toxic meaning poison.

The job of chemotherapy drugs is to kill cells. They are effective against cells that divide rapidly. Normal cells limit their division. Cancer cells, having lost that ability, keep on multiplying and growing.

The skin and the digestive system are designed to self heal which is why their normal cells multiply at a higher rate. Even though they may be healthy they will be affected by chemotherapy. When I talk about the skin with regard to chemotherapy, I include hair and nails. When I refer to the digestive system I include the inside of the mouth and the stomach.

Chemotherapy is administered in order to eliminate the tumor, to reduce the tumor size so it can be removed by surgery, or to shrink the cancer in order to reduce the tumor's effects. For example the effect of a tumor pressing on a nerve is often pain.

Chemotherapy treatment is given orally as a tablet, intravenously as an injection into the vein or by a catheter into the site of the cancer. The treatment is given in a series of courses where the medication is taken for a period of time, then stopped to allow the healthy cells to recuperate. Treatment can be six months or longer, depending on the cancer.

Side Effects Of Chemotherapy

Note: The side effects listed here are the ones I think you need to be aware of for your practice. There are many additional side effects that are life threatening, like damage to the liver, kidneys and lungs. Side effects have been recorded as many as 17 years after the completion of chemotherapy. The secondary cancer risk is another major problem, as any medication that cures cancer has the potential to cause cancer.

Chemotherapy is the most aggressive drug treatment known and has severe side effects. There is a delayed appearance of the side effects. Side effects will appear when the cells start dying. Tiredness or total exhaustion are common side effects because the body needs all its energy to eliminate the damaging chemicals and to heal. Nausea and vomiting will occur and can be treated with medications.

Chemotherapy affects the blood system. Clotting, known as thrombocytopenia, is a common side effect. On the other end of the spectrum excessive bleeding can also result.

Another result of chemotherapy is that veins can appear darker. It is most noticeable with darker skinned people. This will reverse itself once the drugs are eliminated from the body.

Reduction in the function of the immune system makes it easy for chemotherapy patients to become infected.

Nerve and muscle damage can appear as weakness, loss of balance, pain, tingling, burning or even numbness and loss of sensation in the hands and feet. These effects can last up to one year after chemotherapy has ended. Depression is common. It is a reaction to the chemotherapy, the cancer itself and fear of death.

Skin Reactions

Alopecia, the loss of hair from the scalp and from the entire body including the eyebrows and eyelashes, is one of the effects women fear most. Hair will come back once chemotherapy is over. However, it might come back in a different color and or texture.

The nails can become thin and brittle with vertical lines and cracks. They may also become dark or yellow.

Skin will become sensitive, thin and will get infected easily. Skin can become dry, itchy and will be sensitive to sun. Some chemotherapy medications are phototoxic. Preexisting conditions like acne or psoriasis may reappear.

When a patient is receiving chemotherapy the skin site of previous radiation or burn can become red and the skin can blister and peel. This can last anywhere from a few hours to several days. This reaction is called " Radiation recall."

If the chemotherapy leaks or touches the skin where the IV is inserted, pain and ulceration will occur. It might require a plastic surgery correction.

Immunotherapy

Immunotherapy is a new approach in treating uterine cancer. Interleukin or MAbs are used in patients whose cancer has spread.

Salon Treatment

Products containing hormones are not acceptable for women who have had uterine cancer for the rest of the woman's life.

Salon Treatment the First Two Years After Radiation Therapy

CELLS WITHOUT OXYGEN ARE NOT AFFECTED BY RADIATION. WHILE YOUR CLIENT IS GOING THROUGH RADIATION TREATMENT, DO NOT USE ANY OXYGEN TREATMENTS, OXYGEN CREAMS OR OXYGEN BARS. THEY WILL INTERFERE WITH THE RADIATION TREATMENT.

IT IS IMPORTANT THAT YOU DO NOT REMOVE OR TOUCH ANY MARKINGS ON THE SKIN AS THEY ARE RADIATION GUIDES.

While undergoing radiation therapy the patient is highly advised to consult only the treating physician or nurse about skin care, including the type of soap, lotion, powder, deodorant or even sunscreen to use. The skin needs to be protected from the sun, but sunscreens can interfere with the effectiveness of the radiation. The physician needs to be consulted about the use of sunscreens.

No hair removal is allowed at the site and no depilatory lotions. If hair needs to be removed, use an electric shaver, but consult the doctor first. As for hair removal on other parts of the body consult the physician first.

It is important to know that only mild liquid cleanser and moisturizer with no heavy metals should be used by the client. Remember the skin is susceptible to infections. Creams or lotions should be water based and should not contain Vaseline (petrolatum or mineral oil) because they can create a barrier that prevents the skin from breathing, trapping moisture and bacteria thus increasing the risk of infection. Silicones like Dimethicone are good ingredients at this stage. Vitamins, antioxidants, oxygen, peroxide, perfume and any irritating ingredient should be avoided because they can interfere with the radiation treatment. No lotion should be applied within two hours of radiation therapy.

Salon Treatment The First Two Years After Radiation Therapy

After radiation therapy ends the use of vitamin E and silicones can be beneficial to the recovery of the skin at the site of the radiation. At this point you're treating skin that has been severely burned. Consult the physician before any treatment. Do not attempt to lighten the skin or to fight the hyperpigmentation. In time it should fade away.

Do not try to erase the radiation site markings because they might be tattoos. Avoid any aggressive treatment and any exfoliating or antiaging treatment anywhere on the body. Recommend supportive skin care and sun screen. Clients who have undergone radiation treatments are more susceptible to skin cancer. The site of the radiation can be sensitive for a long time. Be careful when treating the skin in that area. In some patients a chronic skin reaction may occur at the site of radiation after six to twelve months. The skin will be thin and easy to break or irritate. Scar tissue may develop under the epidermis. Permanent loss of hair at the site of treatment may occur.

Salon Treatment Two Years Or More After Radiation Therapy

If no other health conditions exist you can resume regular treatments two years after radiation treatment ends. Radiation patients are more prone to develop skin cancers so you need to monitor this client for any skin lesions or skin changes. Please see the Skin Cancer Chapter.

Finally, as the population ages, you will be treating more and more people who have undergone radiation therapy. Now is a good time to get involved with the cancer center in your area. You might be able to work with the nurse or doctor in providing skin care to their patients.

Salon Treatments For Chemotherapy Clients
While on chemotherapy and up to 2 years post treatment.

Before treating this client check with her treating doctor.

Patients are urged by their medical care givers to continue their normal life as part of the overall goal of maintaining a positive attitude to fight and overcome the cancer.

If you choose, you can get involved with your local cancer treatment center and become an integral part of the cancer support system.

Your salon or spa can become a place of refuge and provide a bit of normal routine in a crisis situation. Here are some do's and don'ts.

DO use extra precaution because these clients tend to get infected easily. Avoid any service with the potential to compromise the skin's integrity: like extraction, deep cleaning, hair removal by waxing, sugaring, threading or tweezing.

DO use only clean products and pay special attention to prevent cross contamination.

DO use a mouth mask, especially if you have been near anyone who is sick or with a cold.

DO use products that are gentle, preferably without perfumes and alcohol.

DO use moisturizing creams and lotions, the skin is dry and thin. Some beneficial ingredients are starches from oatmeal, rice or corn, silicones like Dimethicone, Aloe Vera, chamomile, and zinc oxide.

DO recommend a good sun screen of at least SPF 15.

DO recommend a nail strengthener and administer a hand moisturizing treatment with warm oil. Olive oil and almond oil are beneficial.

DO help your client to get off the treatment table to prevent any falls.

DON'T peel or exfoliate the skin. Do not use chemical or botanical/ organic ingredients that thin the skin including AHA, BHA, vitamin A or C. Do not use microdermabrasion or scrubs.

DON'T use any ingredients that have the potential to be absorbed into the skin.

DON'T use any heating masks or extreme cold treatments

DON'T use body treatments like body wraps and massage of the legs because of the risk of blood clot.

DON'T suggest or recommend any oral vitamins , food supplements or any herbal remedies

DON'T use essential oils.

Make Up:

Because of hair loss, including eyebrows and lashes, your client might need your help. You can teach her how to enhance her appearance, but do not use any permanent make up. Because of the danger of infection, remind her to start with new make up and brushes. Recommend products that are water soluble, easily removed with water, containing titanium dioxide.

Salon Treatment Two Years After Chemotherapy Is Completed.

If there are no other conditions you can treat the skin as needed. Remember even after 2 years, the skin can be extremely sensitive and thin. Monitor this client for skin changes as secondary cancer may occur with chemotherapy.

CALL THE TREATING PHYSICIAN BEFORE YOU ADMINISTER ANY SALON TREATMENT TO A CANCER PATIENT, A RECOVERING CANCER PATIENT, OR A FORMER CANCER PATIENT.

CHAPTER 7

Ovarian Cancer

Ovarian Cancer

In the United States more women die from ovarian cancer than any other gynecological cancer. More than 23,000 new cases were diagnosed in the year 2000, and 14,000 women died from the disease. One in every 57 women will get the disease. Although most cases occur in women over the age of 50, it can also strike younger women.

There are two problems with ovarian cancer. The first is diagnosis. Ovarian cancer is very hard to diagnose because in the early stages it is almost symptom free. When symptoms do appear, they are the result of the cancer having spread to other organs.

The second problem is difficulty with early detection which, with cancer, is the key to survival. There is no one test that can detect the disease. The existing tests have a high rate of false positive results often leading to invasive, painful exploratory tests.

The common diagnostic tools used to detect ovarian cancer are pelvic exams where a mass or a change in the ovaries can be felt, a transvaginal sonography (ultrasound) or a blood test for the marker C-125. Although all the tests have a high false positive rate, it is important to have them done annually if the woman is in a high risk group.

C-125 is an antigen that is found in the serum (blood test) when cancer is present. The cancers that cause C-125 to elevate are: ovarian, cervical, breast, endometrium, fallopian tube, pancreas, lung and colon.

Conditions that are noncancerous can also cause elevation of C-125 like pregnancy, endomitriosis, inflammation of the pelvis, and fibroids in the uterus. In addition, about 1% of the female population has elevated C-125 without cancer. C-125 is elevated in 80-85% of all women with ovarian cancer.

The only absolutely positive diagnostic method is surgery, where the abdomen is opened (laparatomy). If a cancer is suspected, the entire ovary is removed to prevent the spread of cancerous cells.

The ovaries are responsible for two very important functions. One is the monthly production of an egg, and the other is releasing the female hormones estrogen and progesterone. There are two ovaries in the female body which are located in the pelvic cavity on each side of the uterus, below the fallopian tubes. They are little, almost flat sacs, no larger than an almond . The ovary is covered with a layer of epithelium type cells. It is a continuous layer that gets ruptured every month at ovulation when a mature egg is released. Under that layer, there is a layer of connective tissue called the stroma and in the stroma are the follicles (germ cells). There are about 400,000 follicles in a young woman, and every month 5 to 15 will start maturing, but only one will come to full maturity and will rapture to release the egg.

Types of Ovarian Cancer

There are three types of ovarian cancer—the epithelial, stromal and germ cell. Germ cell cancer is developed in the egg cell itself; stromal is the cancer of the ovary's supportive tissue. Both are rare. and this chapter does not cover them.

Epithelial carcinoma is the cancer of the surface of the ovary. When the cancer grows, cells separate and move in the abdomen to other organs, then they start growing on the new organ. Most commonly ovarian cancer spreads to the closest tissues and organs like the uterus, the vagina, the membrane lining of the abdomen (peritoneum), to the muscle on the top of the abdomen and beneath the chest (diaphragm), the bladder and the rectum. The cancer can also spread through the blood or the lymphatic system to the rest of the body.

Although scientists do not know what causes ovarian cancer, some evidence shows that the less a woman ovulates, the less likely she is to get this cancer. Pregnancy, birth control pills and breast feeding will prevent ovulation and therefore may reduce the risk of ovarian cancer. So will the prevention of pregnancy by a Tubaligation or a hysterectomy. Reduction of fat in the diet may also lower the risk. If a women is at high risk, the removal of the ovaries can be a preventative operation.

Yearly visits to the gynecologist for a pelvic exam and transvaginal ultrasound are at this point the only early detection methods. A yearly C-125 blood test is controversial.

Risk factors
Age

The older the woman, the higher the risk. Most cases of ovarian cancer occur in women over 60.

Fertility and Fertility Drugs

If a woman is childless, she is at a higher risk. The risk goes down 10% with each child born. If a woman uses fertility drugs to induce ovulation, her risk increases.

Hormonal Replacement Therapy or HRT

There is some evidence that HRT increases the risk slightly.

Talc

The use of talc in the vaginal area for a long periods of time may increase the risk.

Genetics

About 5% of all ovarian cancer patients have a family history of the disease. The regular rate of ovarian cancer in the population is 1.6%. A woman who has a first degree relative, that is a sister or a mother, who had ovarian or breast cance increases her risk three times. If a woman has two first degree relatives, for example, her mother and a sister, she has a 50% greater risk of ovarian cancer.

Personal History

If a women has a defective gene BRCA -1 or 2 she has a 50% risk over a lifetime. Breast or colon cancer in the past will increase the risk of ovarian cancer.

Medical Treatment

Treatment depends on the stage of the tumor, its size and where it has spread. The surgeon will try to remove the entire tumor or reduce its size, so there is less tumor to be treated with chemotherapy and radiation.

If the patient is a young, pre-menopausal woman, the ovaries will be removed, immediately causing the onset of menopause. This is because the ovaries, the organs that produce estrogen and progesterone, are removed.

Hormonal Replacement Therapy

Hormonal Replacement Therapy might stimulate cancer growth. This is why those patients will not receive HRT, and consequently will suffer the side effects of menopause. They will experience hot flashes and the skin will go into early aging process.

Radiation

Radiation is done by an external source or by a catheter inserted into the treated area delivering radioactive liquid directly to the site. Radiation therapy is based on the knowledge that living cells exposed to high energy will be damaged and not be able to multiply. The second fact that makes radiation therapy work is that cancerous cells multiply at a higher rate then normal cells. The result is that radiation is able to damage the rapidly multiplying cancerous cells while limiting the damage to healthy cells.

There are different types of radiation therapy. The most common one is from an outside source. The energy used is X-ray, cobalt-60 gamma ray, electron beam, neutron beam, or proton beam. The beam is directed at the tumor site on the body. The treatment is given every day for several weeks. The time of the exposure is short to minimize damage to the surrounding healthy tissue. If the patient's overall health allows it, she can go home and continue with regular activities when the treatment is concluded.

Remote Brachytherapy is another type of radiation treatment which is done with an outside source of radiation that is directed through a catheter or tube directly to the tumor. This is considered an inside therapy as the beam is delivered directly into the tumor.

Another type of internal radiation is when the source of energy is implanted inside the tumor or in the area where the tumor has been removed.

A variation of this treatment is when the source is not encapsulated but the radioactive material is injected into the body. Since the radioactive material is in the body, the patient is radioactive and needs to be isolated in the hospital. Visitors and medical personal are limited to short visits so they will not be affected by the radiation.

Side Effects of Radiation

Lack of energy is the most noticeable side effect of radiation therapy because the body is trying to heal the damaged cells. Nausea, vomiting, change of taste in the mouth and loss of appetite can also occur. Most side effects will disappear with the end of treatment.

Skin Reactions to Radiation

Skin reaction is usually delayed and can be seen after two weeks or longer from the start of radiation because the damage that is done by radiation to the cell is only pronounced when the cell divides. The reaction can vary from red skin, swelling, itching, to dry skin that is scaling. Sometimes the skin will look like it has been burned and might ulcerate. In most cases the skin will get hyperpigmented.

Some people will develop wet skin, particularly in areas were there are skin folds. Since the skin is moist, it breaks easily which increases the danger of infection.

The patient should wear pure cotton and avoid tight clothing. Itching or scratching of the irritated skin should be avoided at all costs. No heating or cooling of the site is allowed without consulting the treating physician. Do not apply any covering or bandages to the radiated site.

Chemotherapy

Chemotherapy is given by mouth into the vein and in some cases directly into the abdomen (intraepitoneal chemotherapy)

Chemotherapy is the popular name for the treatment of cancer with drugs. This group of drugs is also called Antineoplastic agents: anti meaning against, neoplastic meaning cancer. They are also called Cytotoxic: cyto meaning cell, toxic meaning poison.

The job of chemotherapy drugs is to kill cells. They are effective against cells that divide rapidly. Normal cells limit their division. Cancer cells, having lost that ability, keep on multiplying and growing. The skin and the digestive system are designed to self heal which is why their normal cells multiply at a higher rate. Even though they may be healthy they will be affected by chemotherapy. When I talk about the skin with regard to chemotherapy, I include hair and nails. When I refer to the digestive system I include the inside of the mouth and the stomach.

Chemotherapy is administered in order to eliminate the tumor, to reduce the tumor size so it can be removed by surgery or to shrink the cancer in order to reduce the tumor's effects. For example, the effect of a tumor pressing on a nerve is often pain

Chemotherapy treatment is given orally as a tablet, intravenously as an injection into the vein or by a catheter into the site of the cancer.

The treatment is given in a series of courses where the medication is taken for a period of time, then stopped to allow the healthy cells to recuperate. Treatment can be six months or longer, depending on the cancer.

Side Effects Of Chemotherapy

Note: The side effects listed here are the ones I think you need to be aware of for your practice. There are many additional side effects that are life threatening, like damage to the liver, kidneys and lungs. Side effects have been recorded as many as 17 years after the completion of chemotherapy. The secondary cancer risk is another major problem, as any medication that cures cancer has the potential to cause cancer.

Chemotherapy is most aggressive drug treatment known and has severe side effects. There is a delayed appearance of the side effects. Side effects will appear when the cells start dying. Fatigue or total exhaustion are common side effects because the body needs all its energy to eliminate the damaging chemicals and to heal. Nausea and vomiting will occur and can be treated with medications.

Chemotherapy affects the blood system. Clotting, known as thrombocytopenia, is a common side effect. On the other end of the spectrum excessive bleeding can also result.

Another result of chemotherapy is that veins can appear darker. It is most noticeable with darker skinned people. This will reverse itself once the drugs are eliminated from the body.

Reduction in the function of the immune system makes it easy for chemotherapy patients to become infected.

Nerve and muscle damage can appear as weakness, loss of balance, pain, tingling, burning or even numbness and loss of sensation in the hands and feet. These effects can last up to one year after chemotherapy has ended. Depression is common. It is a reaction to the chemotherapy, the cancer itself and fear of death.

Skin Reactions

Alopecia, the loss of hair from the scalp and from the entire body including the eyebrows and eyelashes, is one of the effects women fear most. Hair will come back once chemotherapy is over, but it might come back in a different color and or texture.

The nails can become thin and brittle with vertical lines and cracks. They may also become dark or yellow.

Skin will become sensitive, thin and will get infected easily. Skin can become dry and itchy and will be sensitive to sun. Some chemotherapy medications are phototoxic. Preexisting conditions like acne or psoriasis may reappear.

When a patient is receiving chemotherapy the skin site of previous radiation or burn can become red, and the skin can blister and peel. This can last anywhere from a few hours to several days. This reaction is called "Radiation recall."

If the chemotherapy leaks or touches the skin where the IV is inserted, pain and ulceration will occur. It might require a plastic surgery correction.

After the chemotherapy and radiation treatments are completed a second look surgery may be performed to see if all the tumor is gone. At this surgery fluids and tissue will be collected and biopsied by the surgeon.

Salon Treaments

Salon Treatment of Radiation Therapy Clients

CELLS WITHOUT OXYGEN ARE NOT AFFECTED BY RADIATION. WHILE YOUR CLIENT IS GOING THROUGH RADIATION TREATMENT, DO NOT USE ANY OXYGEN TREATMENTS, OXYGEN CREAMS OR OXYGEN BARS. THEY WILL INTERFERE WITH THE RADIATION TREATMENT.

IT IS IMPORTANT THAT YOU DO NOT REMOVE OR TOUCH ANY MARKINGS ON THE SKIN AS THEY ARE RADIATION GUIDES

While undergoing radiation therapy the patient is highly advised to consult only the treating physician or nurse about skin care, including the type of soap, lotion, powder, deodorant or even sunscreen to use. The skin needs to be protected from the sun, but sunscreens can interfere with the effectiveness of the radiation. The physician needs to be consulted about the use of sunscreens.

No hair removal is allowed at the site and no depilatory lotions. If hair needs to be removed, use an electric shaver, but consult the doctor first. As for hair removal on other parts of the body, consult the physician first.

It is important to know that only mild liquid cleanser and moisturizer with no heavy metals should be used by the client. Remember the skin is susceptible to infections. Creams or lotions should be water based and should not contain Vaseline (petrolatum or mineral oil) because they can create a barrier that prevents the skin from breathing, trapping moisture and bacteria thus increasing the risk of infection. Silicones like Dimethicone are good ingredients at this stage. Vitamins, antioxidants, oxygen, peroxide, perfume and any irritating ingredient should be avoided because they can interfere with the radiation treatment. No lotion should be applied within two hours of radiation therapy.

Salon Treatment The First Two Years After Radiation Therapy

After radiation therapy ends the use of vitamin E and silicones can be beneficial to the recovery of the skin at the site of the radiation. At this point you're treating skin that has been severely burned. Consult the physician before any treatment. Do not attempt to lighten the skin or to fight the hyper pigmentation. In time it should fade away.

Do not try to erase the radiation site markings because they might be tattoos. Avoid any aggressive treatment and any exfoliating or antiaging treatment anywhere on the body. Recommend supportive skin care and sun screen. Clients who have undergone radiation treatments are more susceptible to skin cancer. The site of the radiation can be sensitive for a long time. Be careful when treating the skin in that area. In some patients a chronic skin reaction may occur at the site of radiation after six to twelve months. The skin will be thin and easy to break or irritate. Scar tissue may develop under the epidermis. Permanent loss of hair at the site of treatment may occur.

Salon Treatment Two Years Or More After Radiation Therapy

If no other health conditions exist you can resume regular treatments two years after radiation treatment ends. Radiation patients are more prone to develop skin cancers, so you need to monitor this client for any skin lesions or skin changes. Please see the Skin Cancer Chapter.

As the population ages, you will be treating more and more people who have undergone radiation therapy. Now is a good time to get involved with the cancer center in your area. You might be able to work with the nurse or doctor in providing skin care to their patients.

Salon Treatments For Chemotherapy Clients
While on chemotherapy and up to 2 years post treatment.

Before treating this client check with her treating doctor.

Patients are urged by their medical care givers to continue their normal life as part of the overall goal of maintaining a positive attitude to fight and overcome the cancer. If you choose you can get involved with your local cancer treatment center and become an integral part of the cancer support system.

Your salon or spa can become a place of refuge and provide a bit of normal routine in a crisis situation. Here are some do's and don'ts.

DO use extra precaution because these clients tend to get infected easily. Avoid any service with the potential to compromise the skin's integrity: like extraction, deep cleaning, hair removal by waxing, sugaring, threading or tweezing.

DO use only clean products and pay special attention to prevent cross contamination.

DO use a mouth mask, especially if you have been near anyone who is sick or with a cold.

DO use products that are gentle, preferably without perfumes and alcohol.

DO use moisturizing creams and lotions because the skin is dry and thin. Some beneficial ingredients are starches from oatmeal, rice or corn, silicones like Dimethicone, Aloe Vera, chamomile, and zinc oxide.

DO recommend a good sun screen of at least SPF 15.

DO recommend a nail strengthener and administer a hand moisturizing treatment with warm oil. Olive oil and almond oil are beneficial.

DO help your client to get off the treatment table to prevent any falls.

DON'T peel or exfoliate the skin. Do not use chemical or botanical/organic ingredients that thin the skin including AHA, BHA, vitamin A or C. Do not use microdermabrasion or scrubs.

DON'T use any ingredients that have the potential to be absorbed into the skin.

DON'T use any heating masks or extreme cold treatments

DON'T use body treatments like body wraps and massage of the legs because of the risk of blood clot.

DON'T suggest or recommend any oral vitamins, food supplements or any herbal remedies

DON'T use essential oils.

Make Up

Because of hair loss, including eyebrows and lashes, your client might need your help. You can teach her how to enhance her appearance, but do not use any permanent make up. Because of the danger of infection, remind her to start with new make up and brushes. Recommend products that are water soluble, easily removed with water, containing titanium dioxide.

Salon Treatment Two Years After Chemotherapy Is Completed.

If there are no other conditions you can treat the skin as needed. Remember even after 2 years, the skin can be extremely sensitive and thin. Monitor this client for skin changes as secondary cancer may occur with chemotherapy.

CALL THE TREATING PHYSICIAN BEFORE YOU ADMINISTER ANY SALON TREATMENT TO A CANCER PATIENT, A RECOVERING CANCER PATIENT OR A FORMER CANCER PATIENT.

Book Disclaimer for Salon Treatments

This book is meant to be a general warning guide only. When treating a cancer patient, always check with the treating physician before administering any treatment. Treatments are mentioned as "Don't" or "Avoid" when there is medical or anecdotal evidence that the treatment may cause harm to your client. If there is no treatment warning, that does not mean it is safe. It might mean that at the time this book was written there was no clear medical or anecdotal evidence that the treatment was unsafe or that it was overlooked.

NOTE: Before you administer any treatment to a cancer patient, recovering cancer patient or former cancer patient, check with the treating physician.

Glossary

Adjuvant therapy (AD-joo-vant)
Cancer treatment given after the primary treatment to make it work better. It can include chemotherapy, hormonal therapy or radiation.

Areola (a-REE-o-la)
The area of dark colored skin on the breast that surrounds the nipple.

Aspiration (as-per-AY-shun)
Removal of fluid from a lump with a needle and syringe. Aspiration is done to get a sample of the cells in the lump to be analyzed by the pathologist.

Benign (beh-NINE)
Not cancerous. Benign growth or tumor does not spread to other parts of the body.

Biopsy (BY-ahp-see)
A procedure used to remove cells or tissue in order to check them under a microscope for signs of disease.

Bone Marrow
The soft sponge like tissue in the center of bones that produces white blood cells, red blood cells and platelets.

Carcinoma (kar-sin-O-ma)
Cancer that begins in the skin or in the tissue that lines or covers internal organs.

Cell
The smallest unit of tissues that make up any living thing. Cells have very specialized structure and function and are able to reproduce when needed.

Clinical trial
A research study that tests how well new medical treatment or other interventions work on humans. Each study is designed to test new methods of screening, prevention, diagnosis or treatment of a disease.

Cryosurgery (KRYE-o-SIR-jer-ee)
Treatment performed with an instrument that freezes and destroys abnormal tissue.

Cyst (sist)
A sac or capsule filled with fluid.

DNA
The DNA is the information code of the cell. The DNA contains all the genes or is made of a combination of all the gene pieces.

Duct (dukt)
A tube through which body fluids pass.

Estrogen (ES-tro-jin)
A female hormone. It can stimulate growth of some breast cancers.

Gene
The functional and physical unit of hereditary passed from parent to child. The DNA contains all the genes or is made of a combination of all the gene pieces. Most genes contain the information for making a specific protein.

Hormones
Chemicals produced by glands in the body. They circulate through the bloodstream to specific cells or organs to regulate their action.

Hormonal therapy
Treatment of cancer by removing, blocking or adding hormones.

Hormonal Replacement Therapy (HRT)
Hormones given after menopause or removal of ovaries to replace the normal body production of hormones in women. The hormones used are estrogen and/or progesterone.

Hysterectomy (hiss-ter-EK-toe-mee)
An operation in which the uterus is removed.

Immune system
The body's own defense system against infection or disease.

Invasive cancer
Cancer that has spread beyond the layer of tissue in which it developed and is growing into surrounding, healthy tissue. Another name is infiltrating cancer.

Intravenous (IV)
Injection into the vein.

Laser (LAY-zer)
A device that concentrates light into an intense, narrow beam used to cut or destroy tissue. It is used in microsurgery, photodynamic therapy and for a variety of diagnostic purposes.

Lesion (LEE-zhun)
An area of abnormal tissue change.

Lobe
A portion of an organ such as the liver, lung, breast or brain.

Lobule (LOB-yule)
A small lobe or subdivision of a lobe.

Local therapy
Treatment that affects cells in the tumor and the area close to it.

Lymph (limf)
The fluid that travels through the lymphatic system and carries cells that help fight infection and disease. It also carries waste from the organs and tissues back to the blood stream so they can be eliminated from the body.

Lymphatic system (lim-FAT-ik)
The tissues and organs that produce, store, and carry white blood cells which fight infection and other diseases. It also removes waste from body tissue and cells. This system includes bone marrow, spleen, thymus, lymph nodes and a network of thin tubes that carry lymph and white blood cells. These tubes branch, like blood vessels, into all tissues of the body.

Lymph nodes
Small, bean-shaped organs located along the channels of the lymphatic system. The lymph nodes store specific cells that can trap bacteria or cancer cells traveling through the body in the lymph fluid. Clusters of lymph nodes are found in the underarms, groin, neck, chest and abdomen. Another name is lymph glands.

Lymphedema (LIMF-eh-DEE-ma)
A condition in which excess lymph collects in tissue and causes swelling. It may occur in the arm or leg after lymph vessels or lymph nodes in the underarm or groin are removed or treated with radiation.

Malignant (ma-LIG-nant)
A cancerous growth with a tendency to invade and destroy nearby tissue and spread to other parts of the body.

Mammogram (MAM-o-gram)
An X-ray of the breast.

Mammography (mam-OG-ra-fee)
The use of X-ray to create a picture of the breast.

Mastectomy (mas-TEK-toe-mee)
A surgery performed to remove the breast or as much of the breast tissue as necessary to eliminate cancer.

Menopause (Men -o - pawz)
The time in a woman's life when the menstrual period stops. Another common name is "change of life."

Menstrual cycle (Men-stroo-al)
The cycle of hormonal change occurring monthly in the female body from one menstrual period to the beginning of the next one.

Menstruation: (Men-stroo-AY-shun)
The vaginal discharge of blood and tissue from the uterus occurring approximately every 28 days when the women is not pregnant.

Metastasis (meh-TAS-ta-sis)
The spread of cancer cells from the original tumor to other parts or organs of the body.

Negative
A lab test result that fails to show a positive presence of a specific disease or condition for which that test is being done.

Ovaries
The pair of female reproductive organs that produces eggs and hormones.

Oncologist (on-Kol-o-jist)
A doctor specializing in the treatment of cancer.

Pap Smear
The full name for Pap smear is Papanicolaou smear. The test is named after George Nicolaou (1883-1962), a Greek physician, anatomist and cytologist that developed the test. Pap smears and pelvic exams are preformed by a gynecologist in the office or in a clinic. The doctor inserts a cotton swab moistened with saline, a wooden spatula, or a little brush into the cervix and scraps a sample of the cells that line the cervix. He then smears the sample onto a microscope glass. The sample is sent to a laboratory were a cytologist analyzes the sample. If abnormal cells are found further testing and examination by the doctor takes place. In order to minimize human error and increase

test reliability scientists are constantly improving this test. Women over the age of 18, earlier if the women has had sexual relations, should get a Pap smear every year.

Pelvic Exam
The pelvic exam is the exam where the doctor feels the inside of the female organs and uses a speculum to look and see if there are any changes in the upper part of the vagina and cervix. The doctor can feel any changes to the female organs, the bladder and rectum, including any swelling, inflammation, change in texture, shape or size.

Pathologist (pa-THOL-o-jist)
A doctor who identifies diseases by studying cells and tissue under a microscope.

Photodynamic therapy
Treatment with drugs that become active when exposed to light. These drugs kill cancer cells.

Platelets
The part of blood that helps blood clot at the site of injury.

Positive
A lab test result that reveals the presence of a specific disease or condition for which the test is being done.

Progesterone (pro-JES-ter-own)
A female hormone.

Prognosis (prog-NO-sis)
The likely outcome or course of a disease. The chance of recovery or recurrence.

Risk factor
A condition, habit or inherited trait that increases the chance of developing a disease.

Screening
Checking for disease when there are no symptoms.

SPF (sun protection factor)
A scale for rating the level of sunburn protection in sunscreen products. The higher the SPF number, the more protection is provided. SPF 15 is the minimum level of protection you should recommend.

Stage or Staging
Classification of a cancer according to its size and extent of spread.

Stem cells
The cells from which all blood cells evolve.

Sentinel lymph node
The first lymph node(s) to which cancer cells spread after leaving the area of the primary tumor. Presence of cancer cells in this node alerts the doctor that the tumor has spread to the lymphatic system.

Systemic (sis-TEM-ik)
Affecting the entire body.

Tissue (TISH-oo)
A group or layer of cells that together perform specific functions.

Tumor (TOO-mer)
An abnormal mass of tissue that results from excessive cell division. Tumors perform no useful body function. They may either be benign (not cancerous) or malignant (cancerous).

Ultrasonography (UL-tra-son-OG-ra-fee)
A test in which sound waves (called ultrasound) are bounced off tissue and the echoes are converted to a picture (sonogram).

X-ray
High-energy radiation used in low doses to diagnose disease and in high doses to treat cancer.

References

Books

Clinical Dermatology— A Color Guide to Diagnosis and Therapy.
Thomas P. Habif. Mosby Press. 1996

Drug Facts and Comparisons.
Facts and Comparisons, Inc. 2001

Martindale: The Extra Pharmacopoeia.
The Royal Pharmaceutical Society. 31st Edition 1996

Fawcett: A Textbook of Histology.
Bloom and Fawcett; Saunders Press. 11th Edition

Harrison's Principles of Internal Medicine.
McGraw Hill. 15th Edition 2001

Monthly Prescribing Reference.
C/O Prescribing Reference, Inc. NY. April, 2002

Oxford Textbook of Medicine.
Oxford University Press. 3rd Edition, 1996

The Pharmacological Basis of Therapeutics.
Goodman and Gilman. McGraw Hill.10th Edition, 2001.

Steadman's Medical Dictionary.
Williams and Wilkins. 24th Edition

Color Atlas & Synopsis of Clinical Dermatology Common & Serious Diseases.
Fitzpatrick Johnson Wolff Suurmond.Mc Graw Hill. 2001.

Dermatology Secrets In Color.
Fitzpatrick Aeling.Hanley & Belfus. 2nd Edition, 2001.

Fundamental Immunology.
Paul Lippincott. Raven

Anderson's Pathology.
Mosby. 4th Edition, 1999.

Clinical Gynecology Endocrinology and Infertility.
Speroff Glass Kase. Williams & Wikins, Ortho. 5th Edition, 1994.

Management of Common Problems in Obstetrics and Gynecology.
Mishell/Brenner. Blackwell Scientific Publications.3rd Edition, 1994.

Current Problems in Cancer: A practical Approach to the Older

Patient with Cancer.
Volume 25 number 1 Jan/Feb 2001
2001 Year Book of Oncology
Editor in chief Patrick J.Loehrer, Sr., MD Mosby

Magazines and Internet Sources

PCI Journal of Progressive Clinical Insights
(201) 670-4100.
National Cancer Institute Cancer information services (CIS)
1-800-4-CANCER www.nci.nih.gov
www.cancernet.nci.nih.gov www.cancertrials.nci.nih.gov
Women's Health In Primary Care Magazine
Clinicians Group Tel # 973-916-1000
www.womenshealthpc.com
Cancer Prevention and Treatment The Good Health Guide
IN TOUCH PRR, Inc. 877-2IN-TOUCH
Drug Topics: The News Magazine for Pharmacists
800-432-4570
Primary Care & Cancer Prevention Early Detection Follow-Up
Journal PRR, Inc. 631-777-3800
A Guide to Skin Cancers and Precancers
The Skin Cancer Foundation Box 561 New York NY 10156
www.skincancer.org Associations:
American Cancer Society
800-ACS-2345 www.cancer.org
Cancer Care, Inc.
800-813-HOPE www.cancercare.org
Look Good... Feel Better 800-395-LOOK
National Comprehensive Cancer Network www.nccn.org
Patient Advocate Foundation www.patientadvocate.org
Patient-Centered Guides 800-998-9938 www.patientcenters.com
City of Hope 800-260-HOPE www.cityofhope.org